Praise for *101 Baby Hacks*

"New parenthood can be extremely challenging to navigate and everyone needs an accessible pocket companion they can reference to troubleshoot the common issues that surface for newborns. Elina Furman's new book, *101 Baby Hacks*, is a guide for new parents who are looking to soothe their babies through easy techniques rooted in science and ancestral tradition. Packed with accessible illustrations and down-to-earth tips, *101 Baby Hacks* is a go-to guide that should be at your bedside."

—Latham Thomas, maternal health expert and founder of Mama Glow

"Elina's book is a gem. Infancy can be such a challenging time with conflicting information, overwhelm, and exhaustion. But no one can argue how touch, and the lasting and incredible benefits humans earn from physical contact, is a sure thing. In this book, Elina provides parents this timeless method, proven over thousands of years and improved to fit our modern times."

—Siggie Cohen, PhD, child development specialist

"As pediatric occupational therapists, we highly recommend *101 Baby Hacks*. In the overwhelming world of baby products and pointless baby books, Elina's expert advice is grounded in developmental science and breaks down natural techniques that promote bonding and brain growth. The perfect gift for a new parent!"

—Carrie Molder and Jenny Jolley, occupational therapists and founders of On-Track Baby

"Elevate your parenting journey with Elina's ingenious solutions! Discover practical and innovative tips that make life with a new baby smoother and more enjoyable and help you all get more sleep! *101 Baby Hacks* is the ultimate parenthood guide and a must-read for new and expecting parents!"

—Mandy Treeby, pediatric sleep consultant and cofounder of Smart Sleep Coach by Pampers

101 Baby Hacks

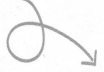

101 Baby Hacks

Infant Massage and Natural Solutions to Help with Sleep, Colic, Gas, Teething, Congestion, and More

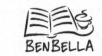

ELINA FURMAN

BENBELLA

BenBella Books, Inc.
Dallas, TX

101 Baby Hacks copyright © 2024 by Elina Furman

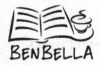

BenBella Books, Inc.
10440 N. Central Expressway
Suite 800
Dallas, TX 75231
benbellabooks.com
Send feedback to feedback@benbellabooks.com

BenBella is a federally registered trademark.

Printed in the United States of America
10 9 8 7 6 5 4 3 2 1

Library of Congress Control Number: 2024007074
ISBN 9781637745373 (trade paperback)
ISBN 9781637745380 (electronic)

Editing by Claire Schulz
Copyediting by Natalie Roth
Proofreading by Lisa Story and Denise Pangia
Text design and composition by PerfecType, Nashville, TN
Interior illustrations by Dasha Kurinna. Instagram: @dasha.illustration
Cover design by Sarah Avinger
Cover image © Adobe Stock / New Africa
Printed by Lake Book Manufacturing

Special discounts for bulk sales are available. Please contact bulkorders@benbellabooks.com.

To my beautiful boys, Julian and Dylan. Forever my babies.

Contents

Coughs, Sniffles, Snots—Oh My! 13 Hacks for Baby Colds, Infections, and Immunity 140

Foreword

As a board-certified pediatrician with a deep appreciation for holistic approaches to health care, it brings me great joy to introduce this invaluable resource on baby massage by Elina Furman. My family immigrated to the United States from India, and my work in pediatric medicine has been greatly influenced by the rich traditions of touch therapy and Ayurvedic medicine in South Asia, where the power of touch is revered for its profound healing properties.

In India, the tradition of baby massage is cherished and deeply ingrained in the cultural fabric, with grandmothers often taking on the role of nurturing caregivers during the postnatal period. For generations, Indian grandmothers have passed down the art of baby massage, imparting their wisdom to new mothers and love to newborns through gentle touch. As a testament to the profound bond between generations, it was my own mother who lovingly performed baby massage for my children. This intimate ritual not only provides physical benefits for the baby but also serves to create a sacred bond between caregiver and child, fostering a sense of connection and security that transcends time.

As a pediatrician and Indian immigrant, I believe in blending the best of East and West to provide holistic care. Preventative and lifestyle medicine focus on addressing root causes and promoting well-being from the start. Unlike medications that treat symptoms, these approaches prioritize prevention, laying the foundation for lifelong health. By emphasizing life-style practices like nutrition, exercise, stress management, and sleep—the latter two of which baby massage can promote from a child's earliest days!—we empower children to thrive and prevent chronic diseases later on.

But parents are up against some challenges.

These days, harmful chemicals seem to lurk in every corner—in the foods we eat, in packaging and plastic dishes, in body products, the list goes on. Many of us are increasingly seeking simple, practical tools to keep our children healthy. Natural solutions that avoid these chemicals in daily products or our food system can be a game-changer in a parent's toolkit. That's why I eventually left clinical medicine to practice preventative medicine at scale—launching Ahimsa, a line of stainless steel foodware made from safe, reusable materials to support healthy eating habits from the beginning. I've been so personally gratified to watch countless families and schools transform their dinner time into a Mindful Mealtime and their lunchrooms into Conscious Cafeterias that nourish growing brains and bodies while protecting the one planet we all call home.

It was on this entrepreneurial journey that I first crossed paths with Elina, in a group for female founders. Her passion for promoting the health and well-being of infants through nurturing touch resonated deeply with me, and I knew immediately that her work with Kahlmi was making a significant impact on the lives of families worldwide. In a fast-paced culture where technology often takes precedence over human connection, the importance of baby massage cannot be overstated. This ancient practice not only provides natural solutions for common infant ailments but also fosters a deep sense of connection and security between caregiver and child.

Elina has been instrumental in helping parents and caregivers harness the power of touch to promote bonding, relaxation, and overall wellness in their little ones. Through her work in baby massage and her and her brand's presence on social media platforms, she has touched the lives of countless families, empowering them with the knowledge and skills to provide nurturing care for their babies.

101 Baby Hacks continues Elina's mission, educating and empowering parents on solutions that have been used for generations in the East. Drawing from the wisdom of ancient traditions, the author provides insights into holistic approaches to wellness that prioritize natural remedies and safe practices that are still in line with the world of modern medicine. By sharing time-tested methods and advocating for healthier alternatives, Elina equips parents with the knowledge and confidence to make informed choices for their children's well-being.

This book serves as a comprehensive guide for parents and caregivers who are eager to learn about the benefits of baby massage and incorporate this nurturing natural practice into their daily routine. From soothing techniques for colicky babies to gentle strokes for promoting sleep and more, Elina offers practical advice and heartfelt encouragement to readers on their journey toward fostering a loving and healthy bond with their little ones.

As you embark on your own journey as a parent, remember that the power of touch is not just a simple gesture—it is a profound expression of love used over generations. By embracing these time-honored practices, you are not only nurturing your child's physical well-being but also fostering a deep emotional bond that will endure throughout both your lives. While you are providing comfort and relief to your little one, you are also carrying forward a legacy of care and connection that spans generations. So, cherish each moment spent nurturing your child through the gentle art of massage, knowing that you are contributing to their holistic growth and development in immeasurable ways.

Manasa Mantravadi, MD

Introduction

The Key to a Happy, Healthy
Baby Is in Your Hands

As a new mom back in 2008, I often wondered: Why can't babies come with an owner's manual!? I'm guessing that, as a new or expecting parent, you may feel the same. So much gets thrown at us so fast. In those early days, I googled everything and anything in hopes of helping my baby:

- Can I cure my baby's congestion?
- Will my baby ever poop?
- Why won't this baby stop crying!?
- Will my baby ever sleep?
- Is there a magic off button that will instantly soothe my baby?

The answer to these questions is, thankfully, yes! For every ailment, issue, and "glitch" our babies experience, there is a natural and simple solution that can help parents alleviate much of the stress of new-baby parenting. Even better, you don't need to shell out big bucks for a robotic bassinet or a bunch of other single-use gadgets. It turns out that, usually, there's a simple massage technique, a useful acupressure point, or another hack that can help you to soothe your baby, ease their discomfort, or help them grow. And in this book, you'll learn a lot of them—101 of them, to be exact. So while there's no owner's manual for an infant, consider this your crib-side companion to hands-on "fixes" you can try when challenges arise.

It feels like forever since my two boys (now 15 and 10) were babies, but I still vividly remember those early, anxiety-filled, sleep-deprived days. The mental fogginess, the stress, the feeling of pure shock that the hospital would even let me take a baby home knowing as little as I did. I've come a long way since then—but if you feel like you're the only parent who hasn't got it all figured out, know that you are definitely not alone.

How a Clueless New Mom Became a Baby Expert

Today, I can proudly call myself a baby expert on social media and TV. As a certified infant massage instructor and the founder of the Kahlmi baby massage company, I now spend my days helping anxious new parents navigate all the issues, questions, and freak-outs that having a new baby entails.

While I may seem to know everything and anything about babies, I was actually the most frazzled, clueless first-time mom I know. I also struggled with anxiety issues and am still dealing with symptoms of postpartum stress disorder years later.

With the arrival of my first son, I quickly realized that I was not adequately prepared for any of it. You might think that, as a writer, I would have read a parenting book or at least some articles to prepare. But I thought that somehow motherhood would come naturally to me. Aren't we taught that women just have innate maternal and caring instincts? I was convinced that pregnancy would be the hardest part of my journey and that my baby would sleep, feed, and thrive on command with little to no intervention.

Instead, I found myself working full-time at home and tending to the immediate and very loud needs of my beautiful but colicky son. He was either crying or eating—just like his mom. As a busy magazine editor and author with my own freelance business, I had to return to work almost immediately after birthing my babies and, like many moms, I did not receive the support I needed. I had the privilege to work from home, but I felt stressed, overwhelmed, and more isolated than ever. I would spend hours researching how to help cure his colic and get him to sleep, all the while trying to deliver for my clients as if nothing had changed. My husband took a week off (so much for paternity leave) and then it was just me, all alone at home with a colicky baby and a mountain of deadlines. The first year of my son's life took an enormous toll on me, not only because of the brutal rigors of being a first-time mom and working from home, but because I had no idea how to manage the ins and outs of baby care and the myriad concerns that "pooped" up each day. It's no wonder I suffered from postpartum depression and anxiety in the first 6 months. I was lost and confused and never expected that I would have such a hard time transitioning into motherhood.

Now that I know what I do, I wish I had learned then about the role that touch and massage play in establishing the connection between mom and baby. I had no idea that learning some basic massage techniques could help both me and my babies thrive. I wouldn't find out about that for several more years—when my oldest son was diagnosed with clinical anxiety. To help support him, I started researching anxiety and children, and I stumbled across the concept of baby and child massage. This holistic, natural practice is performed all around the world and has many benefits for baby's health and development (more on those later), and when it's performed regularly it is just as enjoyable, therapeutic, and relaxing for the parent as it is for the baby.

I began using massage at night to help my son sleep. The difference in him was immediate. I saw improvements in not only his sleep and mental health but also my own mood and outlook. I was surprised to realize how calm and centered *I* felt after each session. I found myself looking forward to our winding-down bedtime routine instead of dreading it. I incorporated massage into our everyday nighttime schedule and would sing songs and tell stories during the massage time to bring us closer together. He tells me to this day how much he loved that time together and still asks me to massage his back as a teen.

Years later, when my son turned 10, I received my certification as a baby massage instructor from the World Institute for Nurturing Communication and set out to create a new brand, Kahlmi (pronounced calm-ee), in hopes of promoting baby massage education and raising awareness to give parents a way to improve their parent-child bond and help nurture their children naturally. In 2022, I designed and developed the first ever baby massager and massage products, which won an iF Design Award, a JPMA Innovation Finalist Award, and the 2024 *Parents* magazine "Best for Baby" award. Now, I'm known as a leading expert on baby massage with over 1.1 million followers on social media.

Ancient Traditions Meet Modern Practices

In India and other non-Western countries, baby massage is considered the *most* important practice of baby rearing. Many families even hire "ammas," women who make daily house calls to perform massage. The practice is deeply rooted in Eastern cultures and is passed down from generation to generation, mother to mother. And yet, in the United States, few parents know about the benefits of baby massage. (There is so much wisdom from ancient cultures that people in the US, and the medical community here, are still trying to catch up on, so don't be surprised if you're late to the party like I was.)

While the practices may be new to many of us in America, baby massage, acupressure, and reflexology have been widely practiced all over the world for centuries. Therapeutic massage dates back to the Ming dynasty in China. It has long been practiced in India, too, as part of Ayurvedic medicine. Other cultures have also practiced these modalities for many years. But it wasn't until the French obstetrician Dr. Frédérick Leboyer popularized infant massage in the 1970s that it started to become more popular in the Western world. Inspired by Leboyer's work, Vimala McClure wrote about the benefits of infant massage in 1976 after returning to the US from an educational program in Indian orphanages.

Beyond tradition, there is good reason why these practices have endured.

When Love, Science, and Nature Connect

Babies are born with billions of neurons. Touch is baby's first sense (our skin is our largest organ), and being touched and receiving massage helps their brains form the synapses (neural connections) that stimulate their development. That means the more you interact with your baby through massage, cuddling, singing, and playing, the more their synapses get activated, leading to improved outcomes for both your baby and you. The first 3 years of your baby's life are critical to their future well-being and will form the majority of their neurological blueprint for the rest of their lives. Clinical studies have shown that baby massage can have an immediate and lasting impact on children's social, neural, and cognitive development. I could fill a book just writing about the science, but you aren't here for that! Still, here are a few highlights.

In the US, Tiffany Field, PhD, a pioneering researcher in infant massage, has been doing studies on premature babies since the early 1980s. But it wasn't until 1992, when she was able to launch the Touch Research Institute at the University of Miami School of Medicine, that baby massage research began in earnest. Field and her team of researchers found that baby massage helped preemies gain more weight than their peers who didn't get massaged. It decreased babies' irritability and crying. It also led to better sleep—both falling asleep faster, and staying asleep with fewer disruptions. "Just adding massage makes such an incredible difference," Field has said. "In everything we've done, massage is significantly effective . . . Massage works because it changes your whole physiology."

The American Psychological Association used Field's research to show that the improvement in growth for preemies resulted in a cost savings of $3,000 per hospital stay. Just talking about economics alone, if the nearly

400,000 premature infants born in the US each year received massage therapy, we would save billions in total health care costs.

More recently, one study out of Bangladesh followed 497 preterm babies who were given daily massages. The researchers found that this ancient practice was not only beneficial, but that it could also save lives: It helped to strengthen babies' skin, improved thermoregulation, and reduced mortality by almost a third.

Today, due to an increase in funding for clinical studies showing the benefits of baby massage for children and families, interest in the baby massage practice continues to grow. Current medical research shows many benefits to massage for babies and children (not just preemies), including:

- Bonding with parents and caretakers
- Physical growth and weight gain
- Regulation of stress hormones
- Longer and deeper sleep
- Reduction in crying and restlessness
- Improvement of digestion and colic symptoms
- Motor development
- Stronger immunity
- Alleviation of pain
- Improvement of jaundice

In addition to all of these benefits, infant massage can help with more day-to-day concerns: helping to get things moving when a baby is constipated or can't pass gas, relieving congestion, and more.

While more and more people are believers in these holistic practices, others think that baby massage is a whole load of bunk. I can't tell you how many times someone on social media has DMed me or commented on one of my posts, "Wow! This can't possibly work!" But even if one massage session doesn't help your baby poop immediately or get rid of their hiccups in an instant, at the very least you will have connected with and bonded with your baby that day.

What's more, baby massage is the one practice that is equally as beneficial for the person giving the massage as the one receiving it. Besides lowering cortisol (a stress hormone), baby massage increases oxytocin, dopamine, and serotonin (known as the "feel good" hormones) in both baby and caregiver. Research has found that giving infant massage leads to a reduction in postpartum depression and anxiety for caretakers. All of this leads to happier, more contented families that have a deep understanding of each other. After all, baby massage is two-way communication. Touch is your baby's first language and allows you to learn all about their likes and dislikes. When so much is competing for parents' attention, that kind of focused interaction is just priceless. In the end, baby massage is a win-win—and the question for most of us is learning how to do it.

Enter 101 Baby Hacks

As a busy mom of two boys, I know how hard it is to read long baby manuals with in-depth narratives and explanations. "Mom brain" and social media have made us more comfortable digesting information in tiny snippets. This book is organized into sections based on the most common baby "pain points": sleep, feeding, poop/digestion, colds and infections, daily maintenance, and motor development. (Having built a strong 1 million+ following of new parents on social media from all around the globe, I was lucky to have such a large focus group to work with when writing this book! I get dozens of questions every day from confused and frazzled parents, which gives me a keen insider understanding of the most pressing baby issues.) Each hack is covered in a short, easily digestible explanation and how-to. While I couldn't cover every issue—after all, it's 101 hacks, not 1 million and 1 hacks—I know you will find plenty of natural ways to help your baby at the tip of your fingers.

It would be great if this information was readily available at every maternity ward, but unfortunately it's not (yet!) something we can learn from our nurses or pediatricians, or even most of our friends. That's why I wanted to write this book. To create the ideal crib-side companion that will show you quick techniques to troubleshoot issues such as teething, sleep, gas/constipation, congestion, hiccups, tummy-time tears, and more.

While there's no one-size-fits-all hack because each baby has their own preferences, this book provides many suggestions for you to try and find what works best for your little one. All babies are different but ultimately the same, in that they will invariably go through the same issues at different stages of their development. This book can help you to create a daily massage practice that will help your baby easily transition from one stage to the next.

What's more, the solutions and hacks are safe, all natural, and based on a mix of ancient and modern practices that actually work. Every hack and massage stroke in this book is rooted in a holistic and mindful approach to baby care. Don't get me wrong—I am not against a dose of Tylenol or a course of antibiotics when needed—but many of us would rather try a nonmedical intervention first. These hacks can also be used in tandem with other treatments with no side effects. So I am all for these natural techniques that cannot harm and can only help your baby.

Most importantly, when you begin a daily practice of infant massage, you will learn that you are inextricably connected with your baby and will feel more empowered to help them. You'll have hands-on techniques you can try to soothe and support your baby—boosting your confidence, too, and ultimately creating a calmer and happier household. By helping to empower and educate families about the importance of two-way physical communication in an ever increasingly disconnected world, I hope to provide a strong foundation for families built on trust, touch, and love. What more could a baby, and a new parent, want? You are already on your way—and the key is right there in your hands.

Top Massage Questions

Here are the most frequently asked questions I get about baby massage. I hope the answers will help you!

Q. Why do I need to massage my baby? I can't possibly add another thing to my schedule!!

A. Baby massage is often viewed as a nice thing to do, when in reality it's one of the most important things you can do for your baby and yourself. Not only does it help with your baby's social, neurological, and emotional development, it will also help you cope with the many challenges of parenthood and develop a deeper bond with and understanding of your baby. And the great thing is, you don't need to set aside hours or even 30 minutes each day to do it—a quick 5-minute massage is all you need. See the Getting Started with Baby Massage section for more tips.

Q. Do I need any tools for baby massage?

A. You will want to have a quality organic massage oil on hand. I especially love our Kahlmi Calming Baby Massage Oil, made with all organic ingredients, but any organic, edible-grade unrefined oil, like coconut oil or almond oil, can also be great choices.

A cushion, baby lounger, or a soft blanket or rug will provide additional padding, adding more comfort for your baby. A loose blanket is also a good idea in case you want to wrap your baby to keep them warm during the massage.

The Kahlmi massager that I invented is also a great tool that you may want to consider adding to your massage toolkit. It has been shown to help babies and kids with gas, sleep issues, and teething due to the enhanced stimulation it provides with gentle and safe vibrations.

Q. My baby hates massage and squirms/cries every time I try!

A. Can you imagine someone not appreciating a good massage? As much as many of us parents would love for someone to massage us all day every day, you have to remember that every baby is different. Some are more sensitive to touch and need more time to acclimate. In fact, some adults do not like massage either as healing touch is something one has to get used to over time. Massage can also be stimulating for more sensitive babies.

For older babies, you can offer them a teether or a vibrating product to help them relax while you do a hand massage. I like to give an active baby the Kahlmi massager to hold since it relaxes them and they can pop it in their mouth for a soothing gum massage. Another trick is to place a floor baby mirror in front of your baby if you're doing a back massage or to place your baby in a gym like Lovevery's so you can massage them while they explore the mobile and other sensory features.

While there are no guarantees your baby will love baby massage right away, the one thing you know for certain is that your baby will change, not only daily but hour to hour. As they go through different stages like teething and sleep regressions, their needs will change and what your baby hated yesterday they might love today. The key to starting a regular massage is trying to do a little every day and experimenting with different strokes, body parts, techniques, and times of day. Pretty soon they will get used to the routine and even look forward to it.

Q. What is the right age to start baby massage?

A. If you're lucky enough to be reading this book before you give birth, know that you can begin a massage practice day one by laying your newborn on your chest and belly and massaging their back and arms and legs. This will introduce them to massage in the earliest days so they can enjoy all the benefits as they grow older. If you are reading this book and your baby is a little older, the right time to start is now! Baby may need some time to get acclimated to a daily practice.

Q. When should I stop baby massage?

A. This is one of the most common questions I get. My answer is always "Never!" Or, keep going for as long as they will let you. While babies experience phenomenal neural and developmental growth during ages 0–3 years, and thus it's especially beneficial at this age, there really is no end date for when you need to stop massage. Many children and adolescents of all ages can benefit from a daily massage practice to lessen growing pains, develop muscle tone, and allay anxiety and sleep issues.

There are many benefits to continuing your massage practice with your child as they mature. Growing pains, anxiety, attention disorders, sleep disturbances, and even eating disorders can be naturally improved with a regular massage practice. I am fortunate that both my boys (ages 10 and 15) still ask for regular massages, especially when they are anxious or can't sleep at night; it's a wonderful bonding experience at any age.

Today's world is nothing if not complicated. Anxiety is at an all-time high among tweens and teens, and social media isn't doing our children any favors. The stronger a foundation we give them in their early years, the more of a protective layer they will have when facing the myriad of interpersonal, emotional, and psychological challenges that lie ahead. Not only will it boost their physical immunity, it will also make them more immune to many of the pressures of the outside world, knowing that they have a loving connection with you as a strong emotional foundation.

They will also learn how to be more mindful and understanding of the principles of self-care, which has a whole host of benefits including improved focus, self-control, compassion, and academic performance.

Q. How often do I need to do baby massage?

A. As your baby matures, you will want to find an ideal time in the morning and night to do the baby massage. In an ideal world, massaging baby twice a day is the best way to make sure they (and you!) get all the benefits of baby massage—but even three or four times a week is enough to keep it a consistent routine that helps you both. See "Getting Started with Baby Massage," on the next page, for more.

Keep Calm and Massage On!

As a new parent, I was anything but calm. Every time I sat down to relax, my baby would start crying. Or, when I would rock my baby for hours and finally get him to drift off to sleep, he would of course startle and wake up the moment his head hit the breathable mattress. It's easy to think in moments like these that your baby is just out to get you, but as we all know your baby is not trying to manipulate you.

Maintaining your composure and calm during these times is no easy matter, so don't blame yourself when you become agitated or disgruntled. Just take a few deep breaths and remember that being a baby is surprisingly hard work. They've spent months incubating in the soft, safe confines of a mother's belly and the world with all its lights, sounds, and new sensory experiences can be quite jarring.

Getting Started with Baby Massage

The most important message that I hope you take from this book is that there is no right or wrong way to massage your baby. Outside of using too-strong pressure or not listening to your baby's cues (both of which we'll cover here), it's very hard to mess up baby massage as it is basically a more intentional way of touching your baby with love—which is something you do a thousand times a day already.

While many parents are concerned or tentative about starting a baby massage practice, learning baby massage is quite simple and intuitive. Here is a quick guide to help you get started.

The Prep

When's the right time for baby massage? Almost any time of day can work. You can sneak a quick 5-minute massage into your daily routine anytime you're with your baby and they seem alert and happy, whether you're giving them a bath, changing their diaper, or playing with them on the floor. If you're riding in the car with them (and someone else is driving), or they're sitting in the cart at the grocery store, try a quick foot or hand massage. You just need to be consistent—and by that, I mean working in massage at least three or four times a week, trying a little every day to get them used to the feeling. Some parents find it useful to set daily phone reminders to massage their babies, but if that feels like too much, don't sweat it. You can also make it a routine that coincides with a daily habit like changing diapers or taking a bath or as part of a nighttime routine so you won't forget.

You will want to massage your newborn when they are alert but aren't irritable or fussy. If your baby is hungry, crying, or restless for any reason, massaging them will not actually calm them down. It may overstimulate them, causing them to be more distressed. So, if they aren't ready (even if it's the "usual" time in your routine!), try again another time.

When you've chosen your time, take these steps to get started.

1. Take a few long, deep breaths and settle into your body. Imagine you are sitting down to meditate and ease into the experience much as you would for yoga.

2. Remove any jewelry and wash your hands.

3. Place your baby on a blanket on the floor, a bed, or their changing station. Have your chosen massage oil on hand.

4. Verbally engage with your newborn. Place your palms together, and ask their permission: "Would you like a massage?" If they smile and make eye contact, the answer is yes. If they are scrunching their face, crying, and/or arching their back, find another time for massage. Asking for consent from a baby who can't talk yet may seem silly to some, but this actually sets up a lifetime value of respect and body autonomy. It also acts as a massage cue for your baby so that, as they get used to a regular massage practice, they can anticipate what's coming next.

The Basic Baby Massage

Here's a quick guide to help you master the basics of baby massage. You can try these basic massages at any time for bonding and development. We will cover different massage strokes throughout the book, so consider this a primer—more details will come in the hacks.

Arm and Leg Massage: Starting with the arms and legs can often be a good way to begin a baby massage since these body parts tend to be less sensitive. To start the arm massage, lay one of your palms lightly on baby's chest to stabilize them, and then glide the opposite hand from your baby's shoulder to their palm using medium pressure (see the next section). Do this three times, and then switch arms. You will do the same strokes for the legs, from their thighs to their feet. Always massage in the direction away from the heart (so, from shoulder to palm and thigh to foot, and not up toward the trunk) as this stroke is less stimulating for baby.

Tummy Massage: Place a flat palm on top of your baby's belly, avoiding the belly button until after baby's umbilical stump has fallen off (which generally happens by the time they are 1 month old). Stroke their belly by making circles in a clockwise direction using medium pressure.

Back Massage: After massaging the arms, legs, and belly, gently place your baby on their belly. This is also a great opportunity for tummy time. You can now gently rub your baby's back using the same circular motion that you did for their bellies.

Face Massage: Place both hands on your child's forehead and trace your fingers down to their chin. Make small circles on their cheeks from their nose to their ears and tracing down the jaw. To help them sleep, gently stroke their forehead straight across with your index finger.

How Much Pressure?

How to get the pressure just right for baby massage is one of the most common questions I get. Most of the massage strokes in this book will direct you to use light pressure. Think of this as a gentle touch—no heavier than would dent a ripe tomato.

Medium pressure can be thought of as squeezing toothpaste from a tube. Firm pressure can be thought of as kneading a dense dough.

You're the Expert

Throughout this book, I've included space for you to jot down some notes about your experiences massaging your baby. As I've said, there's no one-size-fits-all hack, and you might find your baby likes some of these techniques and not others. Or, you might find ways to combine hacks in a way they can't resist . . . and writing it down will help you find that special maneuver when it's 3 AM and you can't quite remember if it was the Jedi Sleep Trick or the Sleep Button that seemed to work so well the last time. You've got this!

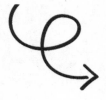

Sweet Dreams
21 Baby Sleep Hacks

Sleep is a universal struggle for new parents. Adults need sleep to function and take care of their babies and themselves. Babies need ample sleep so their brains and bodies can develop. So parents will try just about anything—from robotic rockers and soothing cribs to weighted baby sleep sacks and baby sleep courses—to get their babies, and themselves, some shut-eye. But the truth is, your baby is not supposed to sleep through the night until about 6–8 months of age. As cruel as it can feel to be repeatedly dragged out of bed, night wakings are nature's way of making sure your baby is fed and well cared for even during the wee small hours. The keys to good sleep are getting baby to fall asleep (or back to sleep) faster, and to encourage them to stay asleep for longer and longer stretches.

Some babies are born champion marathon sleepers, only waking up for brief periods to feed or get a diaper change. Others need more help to self-soothe and move back into a sleep state. Now, I'm not here to get into all the different approaches to baby sleep; there are many resources depending on whether you want to sleep train or to adopt baby-led, gentle sleep techniques. But one all-natural and reliable method largely goes ignored: baby massage. While one massage likely won't turn your fitful sleeper into an overnight sleep sensation, studies show that over time babies who are massaged become better sleepers, are more adept at self-soothing, and even produce more melatonin at night.

Baby massage can also be a way to create and maintain a healthy sleeping schedule in the toddler, child, and teen years. Massaging your baby in the evening provides an external bedtime cue that signals it's time for bed. Think of it as a natural sleep cue like books, bath, and bottle. This routine can help to regulate your baby's circadian rhythms and create a more regular sleep pattern, which is vital for establishing a consistent sleeping schedule. Baby massage can also have a calming effect on your baby's nervous system by reducing stress and anxiety levels. Massage can help your baby feel more comfortable and secure by promoting relaxation and reducing tension, leading to a more restful and peaceful night's sleep.

This chapter offers 21 ways to help baby get a good nap or a long stretch of overnight sleep, from massage and acupressure techniques to creating a calm and soothing environment.

Safe-Sleep Basics

The American Academy of Pediatrics has outlined the following safe-sleep basics:

- Always place baby on their back to sleep.
- Use a crib, bassinet, or play yard with a firm, flat mattress and a fitted sheet.
- Make sure there are no items in baby's crib such as loose blankets, pillows, bumpers, or stuffed animals.
- As baby becomes more mobile, and doesn't want to be swaddled, invest in a sleep sack. These go up to toddler sizes so you can feel good knowing your baby is warm and cuddly while staying safe.
- Check baby's temperature to make sure they are not overheating by touching the back of their neck or chest.

Hack #1

The Jedi Sleep Trick

Is baby having a hard time settling? Try the Jedi Sleep Trick to help them fall asleep. Like the Jedis' "mind touch" power in the Star Wars series, getting your baby to sleep is all mind over matter. *The more you believe they will fall asleep, the sooner they will get sleepy.*

Why It Works

The gentle gliding motion of your fingers on baby's face helps calm your baby naturally and creates an almost hypnotic effect. This is very effective with young babies (especially those under 4 months) and works to calm babies after hours of unrest or if they become overtired.

Tips

- Use the Jedi Sleep Trick once baby has settled in for the night after their bedtime routine. You can also lay baby in their crib or bassinet and do this stroke as they are drifting off to sleep.
- To boost the impact, quietly hum or sing a gentle lullaby as they are falling asleep.
- For older babies, the Jedi trick may not work if they are overtired. Try this technique before they become overtired and restless.

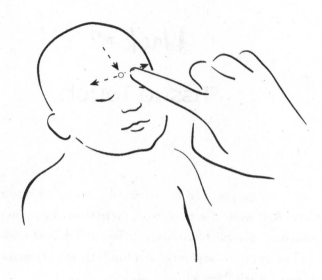

How to Do It

- Using light pressure and just the tip of your index finger, gently glide down from the top middle of your baby's forehead to their brow line. Repeat five to ten times.
- Next, place your thumbs on the inner corners of baby's eyebrows, then draw them out gently to baby's temples. Repeat this stroke five to ten times.
- Move your finger a little faster at first and then slow down your pace as baby gets sleepier and sleepier.

My Notes

_____

_____

_____

Hack #2

Tissue Touch

Can a simple household tissue help your baby nod off to sleep? Yes, it can! And while this won't work every time, depending on how over-tired your baby is, it can't hurt to try. In fact, if it doesn't work and baby still won't fall asleep, it can still serve as a fun little sensory game that can give both of you a laugh. Here's how it works.

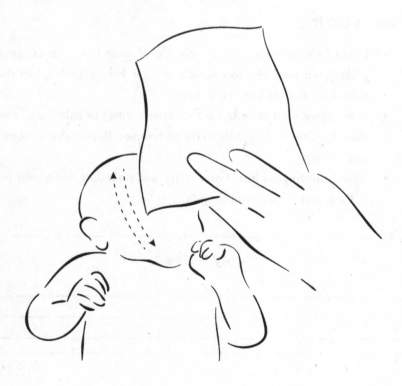

Why It Works

The gentle visual and airflow created by the movement of the tissue helps to calm your baby. By repeating the same motion with the soft sensory feel of the tissue, your baby can settle and relax their visual focus. The motion also helps decrease cortisol (anxiety levels) and settle them in for a good night's sleep.

Tips

- Use a dry tissue, as a wet wipe will just annoy baby.
- Try not to make too much eye contact with baby as this may stimulate them instead of relaxing them.

How to Do It

- To maximize the power of this technique, place your baby in their swaddle or sleep sack (depending on what you are currently using), before you start the tissue trick.
- Take a clean tissue (should go without saying, but you never know) and glide the tissue downward from the top of your baby's head to their chin, barely grazing their face. Repeat the motion by bringing the tissue back to the top and gliding down again from top of head to their chin.
- Repeat the gliding tissue movement five to ten times, slowing down as your baby's eyelids grow heavier. Continue for 2–3 minutes until baby has dozed off.

My Notes

_____

_____

Hack #3

The Waterfall

There is something so relaxing about a head massage. Remember those scalp massagers you used as a kid? It's the same idea, but for this particular hack we will be using the tips of our fingers to create a soothing sensation.

Why It Works

The small muscles around your baby's head and scalp are extra sensitive and receptive to touch. The scalp has even more touch receptors and nerve endings than the back, which means it's super relaxing to have your head massaged. The head and skull also have a lot of stored tension, and massage can help calm and relax your baby.

Tips

- Be careful when massaging baby's skull. Never use strong pressure as they have soft spots called fontanels at the top and back of their head that will need to be avoided. Use very light pressure.
- Softly sing "The Itsy Bitsy Spider" while you do this.
- You could also start doing this stroke while baby is nursing or feeding, right before you lay them in their crib.

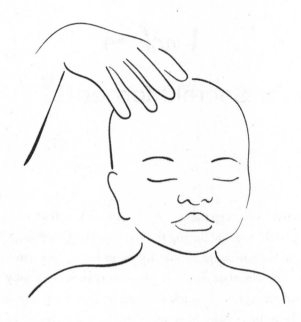

How to Do It

- Place your hands around baby's head. Using just your fingertips and a very light pressure, rub down from the top of their head to their cheeks.
- Repeat for 2–3 minutes until your baby looks like they are falling asleep. Continue massaging your baby's head in the crib, another 2–3 minutes, if they have a hard time settling.

My Notes

_____

_____

_____

_____

Hack #4

Sacral Moments

Massaging baby's back before bed can be an extremely soothing and relaxing experience. And while you will want to do a more invigorating back massage during the day (see the Go, Baby, Go! section), the nighttime back massage should focus on long, slow strokes that calm baby rather than stimulate them. The sacrum is an area on baby's back right at the base of the spine. A quick massage at this point can be extremely relaxing and eliminate pain. Massaging this area and the top of baby's bum can help them fall asleep faster.

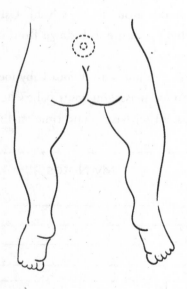

Why It Works

Massaging the back and sacrum helps to relieve pain, hip tightness, and pressure of the spine. It can also bring relief from colic to fussy babies.

Tips

- Always massage the back without pressing on the spine.
- Always support younger babies with a bolster or pillow so they can relax in their tummy-time position.

How to Do It

- Lay your baby on their tummy, with their chest and head on a bolster or a rolled-up towel so they can relax on an incline (this also counts as additional tummy time!).
- Start by placing your palms on baby's back, fingers pointing up, and draw your hands up along their spine and then out to the shoulders, using medium pressure and creating a T shape with your movement.
- Locate the sacrum by feeling gently for the knob right below the spine and make small, gentle circles here; use very light strokes.

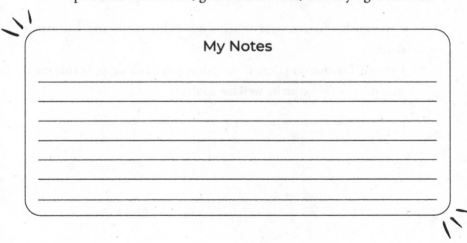

My Notes

Hack #5

Sleep Button

Ever wish there was an on-off switch for baby? Here's the next best thing. This acupressure point is remarkably effective in getting baby to doze off. Called the An Mian points, these pressure points are on either side of the neck right behind the earlobe.

Why It Works

Acupressure is one of the most reliable alternative therapies that can be used for troubleshooting many ailments. The An Mian point relates to insomnia and has been shown to help induce sleep.

Tips

- This can be done several times a day before naps and nighttime sleep.
- Parents: Try this on yourself next time you can't sleep, as this pressure point works equally well for adults.

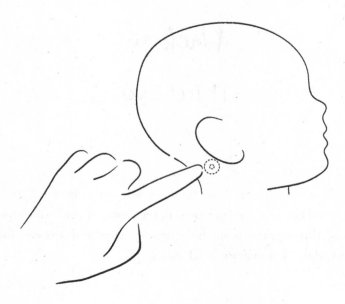

How to Do It

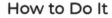

- To locate this spot, place your fingers behind baby's earlobe on one side of their head and move your finger to the soft depression right behind their earlobe.
- Apply light pressure and make small circles. For babies under 3 months, apply pressure for 15–30 seconds. For older babies, apply pressure for 30–60 seconds.
- Switch sides.

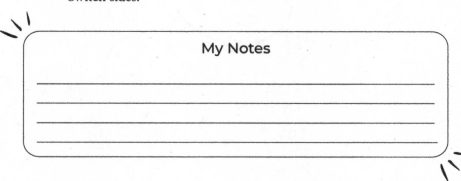

My Notes

Hack #6

Third Eye

The third eye is known as Ajna in Sanskrit. This acupressure point is found between the eyebrows, in the center of your baby's forehead. Massaging this pressure point helps relieve stress and anxiety, improves sleep, and relaxes your baby's facial muscles.

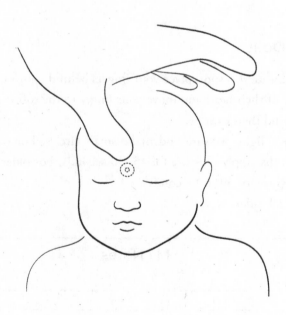

Why It Works

Light pressure applied to the third eye pressure point is known to impact the pineal gland, which plays a role in the circadian rhythm and the secretion of the hormone melatonin.

Tips

- When holding pressure here, play with different speeds and directions, and watch your baby for their reaction (getting sleepier or more annoyed?). Slow down as they fall asleep.
- For older babies, you may want to increase the pressure to medium to help them settle.

How to Do It

- Use your thumb to massage the third eye area located in the center of your baby's eyebrows.
- Alternatively, use your index finger and either keep your finger constantly on the spot or make small, gentle circles.
- Keep the pressure light and massage for 60 seconds.

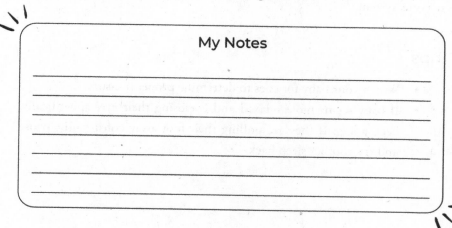

My Notes

Hack #7

Happy, Sleepy Feet

Babies need calming after a morning or afternoon of play. This technique of massaging points on baby's feet is deeply calming and works wonders for soothing and settling an active baby or toddler before nap time or nighttime sleep.

Why It Works

In traditional Chinese medicine, different points on the bottom of the foot correspond to different areas of the body. Activating those points with acupressure—a practice called foot reflexology—is known to help with relaxation and stress relief. By activating points that correspond to the spinal column, this reflexology hack helps calm your baby's parasympathetic nervous system.

Tips

- Watch your baby for cues to determine proper pressure.
- If baby seems more relaxed and is closing their eyes sporadically, keep going. If they are pulling their foot away consistently, pause and try another sleep hack.

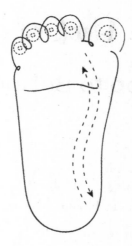

How to Do It

- Hold your baby's foot in one hand.
- With medium pressure, run your thumb along the inside edge of the foot, from the big toe to the heel, then back up.
- Repeat 2–3 times on each foot.

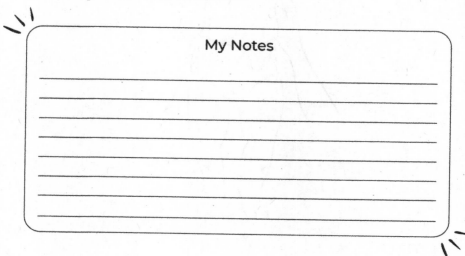

My Notes

Hack #8

Top to Bottom

Babies pick up our energy and laying your hands on them and applying medium pressure can be all it takes to soothe them.

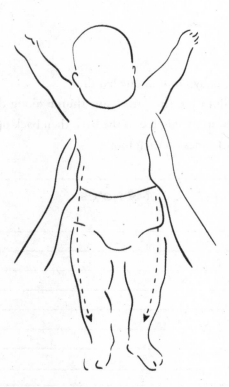

Why It Works

Sometimes just feeling the pressure of your hands can help your baby settle down. Laying your hands on your baby lowers stress levels, boosts oxytocin, and relaxes your baby due to the deep-pressure stimulation it provides.

Tips

- Make a soothing *shhh* sound as you do this.
- Play gentle, relaxing music.
- Use a little organic massage oil to help with the gliding motion.

How to Do It

- Take a few calming breaths so you feel relaxed.
- Position your hands on baby's shoulders and pause for a minute.
- Applying medium pressure, slowly glide your hands down the entire front length of their body to their toes.
- Repeat the same motion but focus your attention on the sides of baby's body, running your hands down the sides of their body, their arms, and their legs.
- Repeat 3–5 times, each time slower than the next to relax your baby gradually.

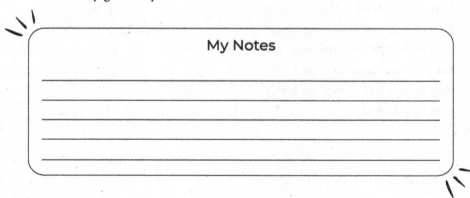

My Notes

Hack #9

Baby-Safe Aromatherapy Massage

Natural edible-grade oils have been used for centuries to help babies and adults fall asleep. After all, they are natural and have strong healing properties to help with a variety of ailments. Essential oils are very concentrated and may be dangerous for your baby even when diluted. The safest oils to use are organic, unrefined, edible-grade oils like coconut, apricot, and chamomile (chamomile helps with sleep). The trick is to experiment and find the right oil that will let your baby fall gently into dreamland.

Why It Works

An oil massage can hydrate skin and many studies have shown that oil massage can help with everything from sleep to eczema, gas, and protecting the skin barrier. Plus, giving your baby a massage with oil is extremely relaxing for both caretaker and baby and allows your hands to glide gently over baby's skin.

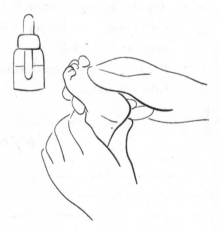

Tips

- Use organic, unrefined oil on baby's body. You can find organic oils that are already diluted that are safe for baby's skin. My brand Kahlmi makes a great organic baby massage oil.
- Only use essential oils in a diffuser for babies 6 months+. Stop use if baby is coughing or showing other symptoms of respiratory distress.
- Never use essential oils on baby's skin as it can cause irritation.
- Massage an organic oil blend immediately after bath to lock in moisture.

How to Do It

- When trying a new type of oil, always do a skin patch test first on your baby to make sure there are no reactions or allergies. To do a patch test, dab a little oil on the tip of your finger and place it behind your baby's ear or behind their knee. Wait 24 hours to make sure there is no irritation.
- Take a little of your chosen diluted oil and massage baby's body. Use only a small dot on the face and massage the chest so baby can inhale the scent.
- Massage the rest of the body using the diluted oil, concentrating on the belly and feet.

My Notes

_____

_____

_____

_____

_____

Hack #10

Wiggle It—Just a Little Bit

Nothing knocks out baby faster than the gentle rocking and vibrations that they feel when riding in the car. Babies have a tendency to instantly fall asleep in a moving vehicle, even after a long nap. And while many parents will pop their baby in the car seat and take a spin around the block to help their baby fall asleep (I can't tell you how many times I was caught driving around the neighborhood), you can recreate the same sensation without ever leaving the house by simply creating a similar wiggle movement.

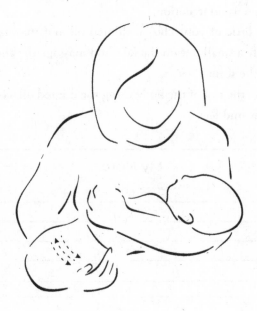

Why It Works

The wiggling motion creates a feeling of a constant vibration and motion that helps your baby fall into a deeper sleep state. Much like the soothing vibrations of a car ride, the wiggling motion creates the same effect that baby felt while in the womb. Also, the confined space within the crook of your arm gives your baby a sense of security and the feeling of being snuggled.

Tips

- Never wiggle too hard or too fast. Watch baby's head as you wiggle to make sure it's just a very slight movement as stronger wiggling can be dangerous for baby. Never shake a baby!
- You can also try this as a different hold with baby's chest pressed against your heart so they can feel connected as they did while in the womb.

How to Do It

- Hold your baby in the crook of your arm, making sure to create a snug feeling as you pull them to your chest.
- With the other arm, start wiggling their bottom gently. As you do this, notice that this will cause their head to gently wiggle as well.
- Continue wiggling for 2–4 minutes until your baby has settled down.

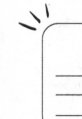

My Notes

_____

_____

_____

Hack #11

Walk and Sit

A recent study out of Wako, Japan, found that a simple, well-timed routine can help your baby stop crying and settle down into a deep sleep. I wish I had known when my kids were little that just 5 minutes of walking followed by an 8-minute sitting sesh can help calm your baby down.

Why It Works

There's a reason this one-two punch works so well. The walking effect is actually called a "transport response" and it is a physiological response that allows your baby's heart rate to slow down when they are picked up and carried. The sitting part has to do with holding them so that their startle or Moro reflex does not activate, allowing them to fall into a deeper sleep before you lay them down in the crib.

Tips

- Use your phone's timer (set to vibrate, not sound!) so you can keep track. Stick to the timed formula exactly.
- Resist the urge to slow down or stop walking to check on baby.
- Don't make any sudden stops or pivots when walking with your baby. Try to keep your stride as smooth as possible.

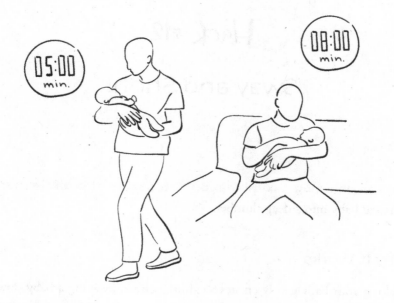

How to Do It

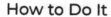

- Make sure baby feels snuggled in your arms, a carrier, or a swaddle.
- Start by slowly walking around the house with your baby, holding them firmly over your shoulder or in a football hold. Walk for 5 minutes.
- Once the 5-minute walking warm-up is complete, sit down and continue to hold your baby for an additional 8 minutes. Lay them down once they look like they are fully asleep.

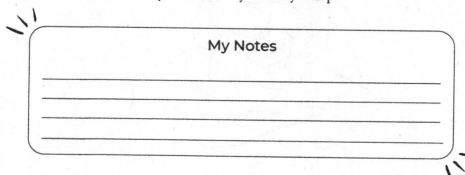

My Notes

Hack #12

Sway and Shhh!

There is one magic combination that can send even the most overtired baby into a deep slumber.

Why It Works

Rocking your baby gently creates a calming effect. Swaying a baby slowly helps to regulate baby's heart and nervous system. The *shhh* sound mimics the sound of being in the womb and helps baby relax and fall asleep.

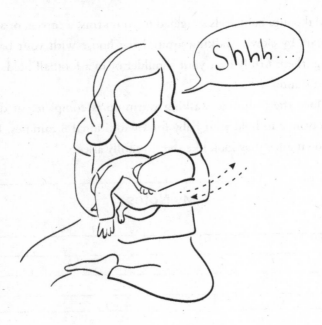

Shhh...

Tips

- Never sway or rock a baby too strongly. Always make sure you are supporting baby's head in your arm or against your body.
- When making the *shhh* sound, make sure to keep your voice quiet if shushing directly into their ear as loud noise could startle them.

How to Do It

- Place your baby in a straddle position over your arms (this position is sometimes called the football hold). Make sure baby's head is lying on your arm and spread out your fingers so their body is fully supported by your palm and fingers.
- Start swaying back and forth gently.
- Add a *shhh* sound as you perform this maneuver.
- Repeat for 5 minutes until baby begins to fall asleep.

My Notes

_____

_____

_____

_____

_____

_____

_____

Hack #13

Butt First! Sleep Transition

One of the worst culprits of baby sleep disruption is the dreaded sleep transition. There's nothing more frustrating than getting your baby to sleep, lowering them into the crib oh so gently and quietly, and then having them wake up screaming bloody murder as soon as you lay them down.

Why It Works

By laying them down with their butt and legs first and slowly letting their head slide onto the mattress, you are preventing the Moro reflex from kicking in, which often creates the sensation of falling if baby's head goes down first.

Tips

- When baby has quieted in your arms, always wait a full minute to see if baby is deeply asleep before transitioning them into the crib.
- Use the other techniques outlined in this chapter to ensure an optimal sleep environment: heat, smell, sound, light, and swaddle or sleeping bag.
- Move baby very slowly to create a seamless transition.

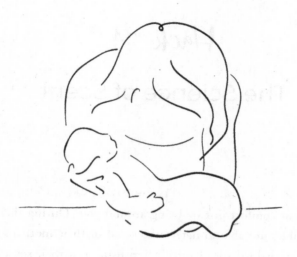

How to Do It

- Many parents place the head down first, but this makes your baby feel like they are falling. Hold your baby closely to your chest and lay their butt and legs down first.
- Once you have laid them down, place a hand over their chest and belly to create a gentle weighted sensation that will calm them. Keep your hand there for about a minute or until baby looks like they are settling.

My Notes

Hack #14

The Science of Scent

Did you know that babies can recognize their caregivers' smell and find instant comfort just by being around you? During their time in the womb, babies are able to detect the smell of their mother's amniotic fluid, which can help them identify Mom using just their sense of smell. If you're looking to transfer baby and help them self-soothe, leaving your scent behind is a great way to comfort them.

Tip

- Never leave anything larger than a washcloth or burp cloth in the crib with your baby.

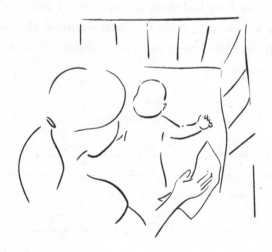

Why It Works

The sense of smell along with the sense of touch are the first senses to develop in utero. Studies show that babies are instantly comforted by their caregivers' smell and presence. When your baby catches a whiff of your scent, they feel as though you are right there with them, which helps ease separation anxiety. A caregiver's scent has the ability to lower cortisol levels, which can lead to deeper, more prolonged sleep.

How to Do It

There are many ways you can capture that magical Mom (or Dad) scent. Try one of the following:

- Place a small cloth in your bra or shirt and wear it throughout the day or during sleep.
- If you're breastfeeding, rub some breast milk on a small washcloth and leave it in the crib with your baby. (While safe sleep rules dictate that you shouldn't leave anything in the crib with your baby, you can leave them with a small 9-inch square washcloth.)
- Sleep with your baby's sheet for a night before laying it down in their crib.
- You can also just rub the T-shirt you wore all day on baby's crib sheet in a pinch.

My Notes

_____

_____

_____

_____

Hack #15

A Warm Landing

Babies lose heat much faster than adults—almost four times faster, actually. One of the hardest parts of getting baby to sleep is to transfer them from the warm confines of your arms to a bare, cold crib. Here's a quick hack that will ensure an easy, cozy transition from arms to the crib or bassinet.

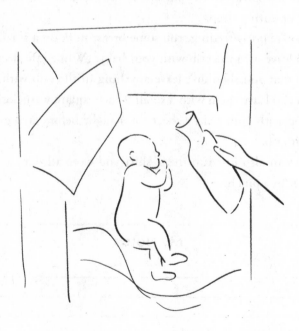

Why It Works

The sudden transition from the warmth of your arms to a colder crib sleep setting can startle your baby awake. A warmed mattress makes it easier for your baby to stay cozy and stay asleep for longer stretches.

Tips

- This can't be overstated: **Never** leave a heating pad in the crib with baby. Always remove once the mattress feels warm.
- While it's important to keep baby warm, also make sure baby is not overheating by creating an optimal sleep environment not to exceed 72°F.

How to Do It

- Place a heating pad (on the low setting) or a hot water bottle in your baby's crib 5–10 minutes before you lay them down. Do a temperature check with your hands. Remove the pad or bottle once the mattress feels pleasantly warm (not hot).
- **Always** remove the heating pad before placing your baby in the crib.
- Monitor your baby's temperature by placing your hand on the back of their neck or on their chest.

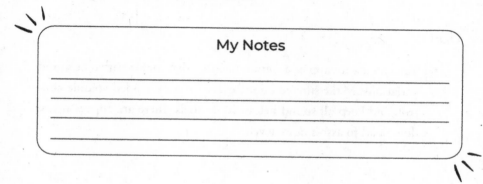

My Notes

Hack #16

Sounds of Silence

While some parents swear by maintaining a noisy environment to get their babies used to sleeping in any conditions, others wouldn't dream of letting their baby sleep without a sound machine at home or on the go.

Why It Works

Ample research shows that certain noise frequencies can have a calming effect on baby's sleep. A 2018 study found that babies who listened to white noise slept more and cried less than babies who were just soothed in a swing. Experiment with different sounds to find out which is most calming, especially for sensitive babies and those with sensory issues.

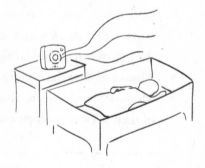

Tips

- You can use an app or a sound machine that makes different sound variations. Make sure you don't exceed recommended volume control, and keep all sound below 50 decibels (there are apps you can download to assess noise level).

- Always place the sound machine 7 feet from baby's sleep area and turn the volume down or shut it off after they have fallen asleep.
- Don't forget to bring your noise machine when traveling and to turn on noise to minimize distractions when entertaining at home.

What It Is

- White noise: White noise mixes sound frequencies across the spectrum, low to high frequency, to make a noise that you might associate with TV static, a fan, or an untuned radio. Most sound machines use white noise as it is most similar to the *shhh* sound that helps babies regulate their nervous systems and relax.
- Pink noise: Pink noise is like white noise but without the higher-frequency sounds, so it can be more soothing to some. It can be compared to rainfall or waves lapping the shore.
- Red or brown noise: This noise color has even lower frequencies, creating a more soothing lullaby-type experience. Think of it as a little deeper than pink noise and similar to the sound of a steady shower stream or heavy rain shower.

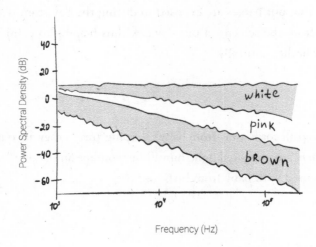

Hack #17

Night-Lights

There are many night-lights available for a baby's room; some are combined with sound machines, some come in fun shapes, others are more simple and plain. Rather than a standard white or yellow glow, try a red night-light for baby's room. It may surprise you, but red light is a natural way to help a baby sleep.

Why It Works

Numerous medical studies have shown that red light therapy is the most natural way to help your baby produce melatonin to help them sleep and regulate their circadian rhythms. It can also offset the energizing impact of blue light that our babies are exposed to during the day from natural sunlight and from the screens of our devices, thus helping to calm them and relax their bodies naturally.

Tips

- Keep all cords away from baby's sleeping area so they are out of reach.
- There are many red light/humidifier combos on the market that can be used with baby from birth on.

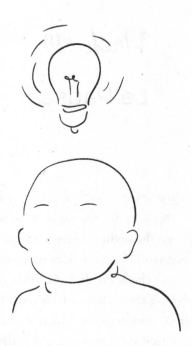

How to Do It

- Place the light source at least 4 feet away from baby's crib.
- Turn on the red light in baby's room while you nurse or massage them to get them acclimated.
- Use the red light every night to create consistent sleeping patterns.

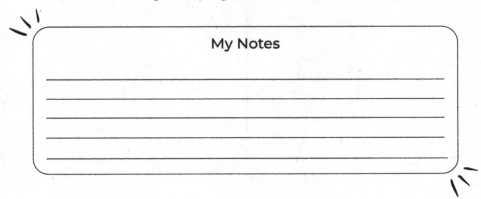

My Notes

Hack #18

Le Pause

Babies are incredibly loud sleepers. Still, not every noise or whimper means that baby is up for the night. One of the biggest reasons babies don't sleep through the night is because we parents have a tendency to disturb them unnecessarily. When babies make noise or start moving, our instinct is to run and check on them but that can actually sabotage their sleep. The French have always been a little more laissez-faire and don't hover as much as their US counterparts, which is where the Le Pause trick comes in. Try this sleep hack next time your baby stirs.

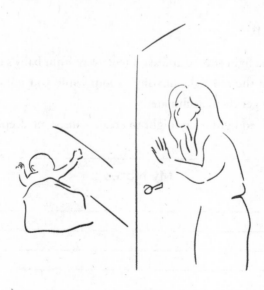

Why It Works

Babies go through many stages of sleep. Sometimes it seems they have woken up, but really they are just passing through different sleep cycles.

The REM sleep stage is frequently called "active sleep" and NREM is called "quiet sleep." During "active sleep," or REM, a baby can be seen making small movements like jerking and twitching so it's important to give them a few minutes to settle.

Tips

- The Le Pause method is not cry-it-out or sleep training. It's simply allowing babies to self-soothe and not interrupting their natural sleep cycle.
- Do not let a baby cry for a prolonged period of time. Check on baby and pat them in the crib if they continue to cry after 2–3 minutes.

How to Do It

- When you hear your baby whimpering, resist the urge to go into their room or wake them.
- Wait 2 minutes to see if they will self-soothe and go back to sleep.
- If they don't move back into another sleep stage, you can check on them then to see if it's a diaper leak or hunger.

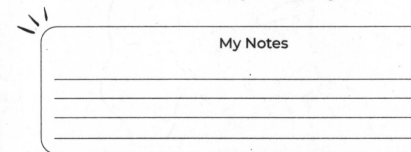

My Notes

Hack #19

Swaddle, Don't Startle

Babies under 5 months have a natural reflex called the Moro reflex that startles them while they are awake or during sleep. While some babies can startle and fall back asleep, other babies often wake themselves up and have a harder time settling back to sleep.

Why It Works

Swaddling prevents your baby from startling themselves awake. The Moro reflex is an entirely natural reflex, and swaddling stops your baby from acting on the Moro reflex to extend their arms and wake themselves up.

Moro Reflex

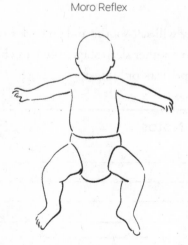

Swaddled Baby

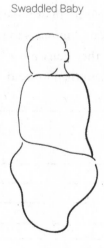

Tips

- The Moro reflex dissipates between ages 3–5 months.
- Make sure you stop swaddling baby when they show signs of rolling over.
- If baby is beginning to show signs of rolling but still likes being swaddled, experiment with one arm out or two arms out, just swaddling their torso. This is also helpful for babies who suck their thumb for soothing.
- Swaddles should always be hip friendly and leave room for movement to ensure proper hip development.

How to Do It

- To keep baby sleeping, try swaddling baby with a traditional swaddle blanket.
- When swaddling, always make sure that the top of the swaddle material starts right below the shoulders so as not to constrict their natural shoulder development or ride up over their face.
- Always place baby on their back when swaddled.

My Notes

_____
_____
_____
_____
_____
_____
_____
_____

Hack #20

Magnesium: The Sleep Helper

Magnesium is a mineral that can be found in foods like spinach, kale, nuts, seeds, and beans. Sleep issues may stem from your baby not getting enough magnesium, which is why I love adding it as a foot rub as part of the nightly sleep routine. Magnesium baby balm or a diluted magnesium spray can be used on baby starting at 7 months old.

Why It Works

Magnesium is one of the most abundant elements in the human body. Magnesium is required for activating enzymes that regulate digestion and boost nutrient absorption, helping the body to function correctly. It will assist in relaxing your baby's nervous system and will improve the quality of their sleep by decreasing cortisol levels that can keep them awake.

Tips

- Only use magnesium on babies 7 months and older. Spray 1–2 times for babies under 1 year old. As they grow, you can increase the dosage to 3 sprays.
- Use sparingly (especially when applied on the feet) so babies don't ingest it.
- Use with toddlers and older kids for growing pains and nighttime restlessness.

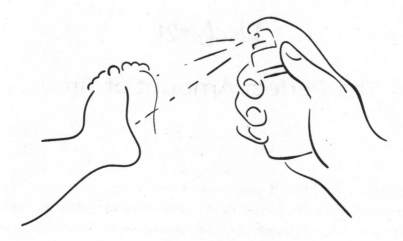

How to Use It

- Get a topical magnesium product made specifically for babies.
- Spray 1–2 sprays or apply a small amount of balm on baby's feet and stomach and massage it in.
- Repeat daily to help baby and kids sleep as magnesium levels build up over time in the body.

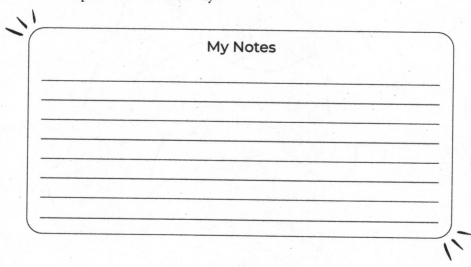

My Notes

Hack #21

The Perfect Amount of Tired

Wouldn't it be nice if you could know when your baby was sleepy so that you can prevent them getting overtired? While your baby can't tell you when it's time to sleep, there are many ways they communicate their level of tiredness with you.

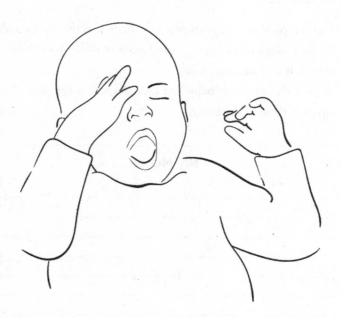

Why It Works

Learning your baby's sleep cues is a very simple process. Babies communicate with us nonverbally all the time, and it's up to us to learn what cues and signals they give us and make sure to follow their wake windows to help them settle into a sleep routine.

Tips

- Three yawns mean it's time for sleep. Wait any longer and baby may be overtired.
- Don't worry if you reach the overtired stage. It happens to all of us!
- Watch baby during their wake windows so you can learn to pick up cues more easily.

How to Identify Baby's Cues

- *Getting Sleepy* cues include long blank stares, flushed eyebrows, and not making eye contact.
- *Need Sleep Now* cues include bigger yawns, rubbing their eyes, pulling their ears, and fussiness.
- *Overtired* cues include prolonged crying, pushing away with arms and legs, and turning the head side to side.

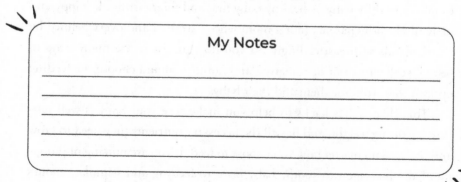

My Notes

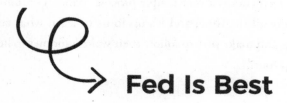

Fed Is Best

20 Baby Feeding Hacks

There are many schools of thought about how to feed your baby. The World Health Organization recommends exclusively breastfeeding for at least the first 6 months and even as long as 2 years. There are many benefits to breastfeeding (immunity for baby, weight loss for mom, bonding, and so on), but many mothers are either unable to or choose not to breastfeed for a variety of personal, health, and social reasons and should never feel guilty for choosing formula. When it comes to formula or breast milk, or a combination of both, the decision is entirely up to each family. While many moms feel guilty if they can't or choose not to breastfeed, I'm here to say that there is no need for that: There really is not one "right" way to raise a healthy baby. A healthy baby first and foremost needs happy and mentally healthy parents (not a mom who is stressed and overwhelmed by the demands of breastfeeding!). So you do you. There are many ways to be an excellent parent or caregiver, and families should choose the feeding options that work for them and their baby.

This chapter has hacks to help you make sure your baby is well nurtured, gaining weight, and has all the necessary nutrients they need to grow and thrive—no matter how you choose to feed. If you are nursing or pumping, baby massage can soothe baby prior to feeding and stimulate mom's production of prolactin, the hormone that helps with milk production. Baby massage also increases mom's oxytocin, which is responsible for milk letdown. And regardless of how you choose to feed, this chapter offers many more general solutions to problems that can crop up with feeding—like oral motor issues, hiccups, reflux, and feeding strikes.

Our motto here is Fed Is Best and, while we all have our plans and preferences, your baby's growth and development is the top priority. So read on for science-supported and all-natural ways to feed your happy little bub. I got you—and you've got this!

Hack #1

Indian Milking Massage

When in doubt, massage it out. While some babies will have no issues guzzling their milk or formula, others need a little encouragement. Performing a relaxing massage before feeding or nursing can help baby relax and calm down, especially if they are older or more active and have a harder time settling. Indian milking is a massage technique that derives its name from this massage stroke commonly used in Indian households.

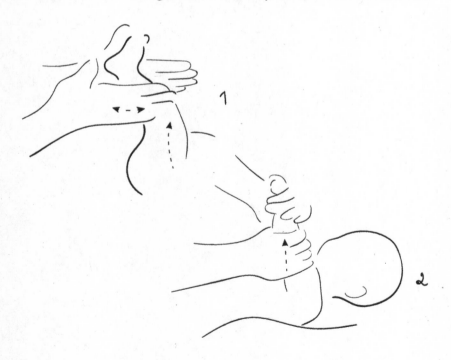

Why It Works

Studies have shown that a calming massage before feeding can help release oxytocin in both mom and baby, and a relaxed baby will settle down to feeding more effectively than an active baby looking to play. Also, if you choose to breastfeed, this massage will help release prolactin, the hormone that increases milk production, leading to a faster, more plentiful flow.

Tips

- Create a serene, non-stimulating environment. Draw the shades, dim the lights, put on soft music.
- Always keep one hand on baby as you work your way down their arm or leg, alternating your hands so one is always connected to baby's leg or arm.
- Take a few deep breaths to promote relaxation as baby will pick up on your energy.

How to Do It

- Curve one hand into a C shape. Support baby's foot with the other hand and encircle the leg with your C hand, slowly milking down from the thigh to the foot with a gentle twisting motion. Repeat three to five times, then move to the other leg and do this on the other side.
- Hold baby's hand with one hand and place your other hand close to baby's shoulder, gliding and twisting your hand in that same gentle milking motion down to their palm. Do this three to five times. Repeat on the other arm.

Hack #2

Guppy Hold

The Guppy Hold is a great technique for feeding or anytime your baby seems fussy for no apparent reason. Used by many chiropractors, this exercise is designed to release tension in the head and neck, while stretching tight neck muscles to make it easier for baby to feed.

Why It Works

Think of the Guppy Hold as reverse tummy time. It allows your baby to extend their chin and stretch their neck, which they rarely get to do. It's very beneficial for building neck strength and will help them feed better.

Tips

- Hold your baby with both hands to support and stabilize them.
- Allow your baby to determine their own level of stretch by letting them take the lead. If your baby gets fussy in this position, draw them closer to you so their head is more supported by your knees.

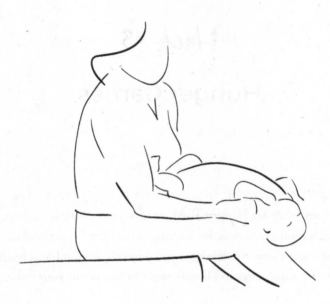

How to Do It

- Sit in a chair in an upright position. Gently place baby on their back on your lap, slowly allowing their neck to extend backward.
- Make sure their head is right at your knees to keep some support for the back of their head.
- Let your baby extend their neck back naturally to stretch their muscles for 1–2 minutes.

My Notes

_____
_____
_____
_____

Hack #3

Hunger Games

For parents of young infants, it can be hard to tell if baby is crying because they are hungry, tired, or just uncomfortable for some other reason and looking to soothe by sucking. (This can be particularly annoying for a nursing mom—sometimes you wind up feeling like a human pacifier!) Here are some ways to identify signs of hunger in your babe.

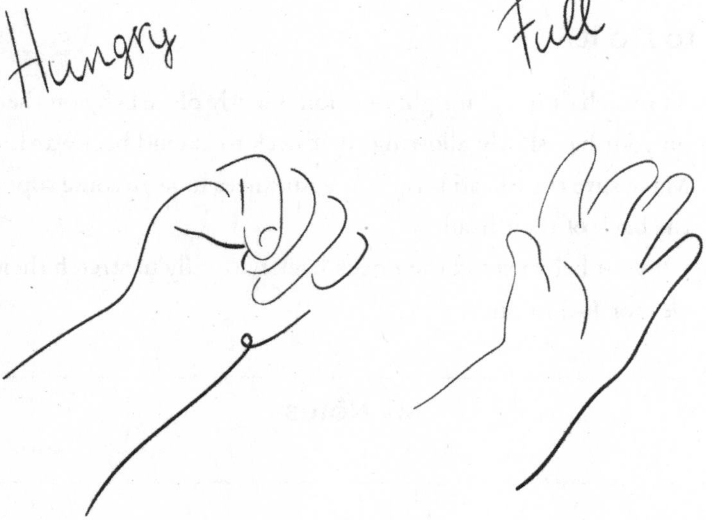

Hungry

Full

Why It Works

Since babies can't verbally communicate with us, it's important to look out for nonverbal cues to understand what they need. By paying attention to these cues, you will learn to understand the signs that your baby is hungry. These can differ from baby to baby and may change at various stages.

Tips

- Not every baby will have the same hunger signs.
- Watch your baby carefully for clues that they are hungry before they become irritable.
- Don't wait to feed your baby when they are already "hangry" as this can make them gassy. If your baby is crying and fussing, try to calm them down prior to feeding.

How to See the Signs

- Closed palms: This is likely a sign that your baby is hungry. If they are crying and their fists are clenched, it may be time to feed.
- Open palms: If your baby's palms are open, this is usually a sign that they are full and satiated.
- Fists in mouth: For young babies, placing their fists in their mouth is usually a sign of hunger.
- Rooting: Turning their head and smacking lips or opening mouth is often a cue that they are searching for something to latch on to.

My Notes

_____

_____

Hack #4

Hunger Strike Busters

There is only one thing scarier than a baby who won't sleep, and that's a baby who won't eat! I can't tell you how many panicked DMs I get when a baby suddenly refuses to nurse or take the bottle. The truth is, feeding strikes are very common, but that doesn't make them any less scary for parents. There are many factors that can contribute to a hunger strike: colds, letdown issues, new perfume, or even parental stress. Eventually every baby will nurse or drink from a bottle, but here are some hacks to help them along.

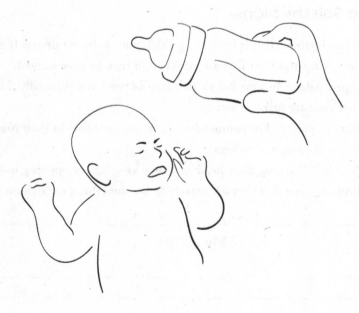

Why It Works

As babies grow and become more active, what worked for them in infancy may not work today. They may need a faster flow or spoon-feeding.

Tips

- All babies will feed eventually. Try not to stress. It's very important that you stay calm.
- You can ask your partner to try feeding the baby as this can sometimes spur your baby to drink.
- Try nursing or bottle-feeding in a quiet, dim room so your baby is not distracted.
- It may be time to introduce solid foods if your baby is 4–6 months old, has good head and neck control, and is showing signs of interest in parents' food.

How to Do It

- If your baby won't nurse or take a bottle, try feeding them with a spoon or feeding syringe to make sure they get some nutrients.
- For bottle strikes, you can try to change up the nipple to see if a faster flow will help.

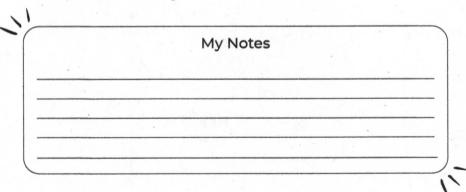

My Notes

Hack #5

Cry Decoder

Did you know you could decode the universal language of babies just by learning to recognize different crying sounds? Crying is actually a very adaptive behavior. While many parents worry when their babies cry, it's actually the best and only way they can communicate with you to let you know they need attention, so try not to feel stressed when you hear baby crying. Instead listen for these cues and respond appropriately:

- "NEH" is the sound baby makes when they are hungry. The sound is created when baby's tongue touches the roof of their mouth, which creates a sucking reflex.
- "OWH" is usually long and drawn out and can mean baby is over-stimulated and sleepy. It kind of sounds like a long "OUCH" without the "CH," with baby's mouth forming an oval shape.

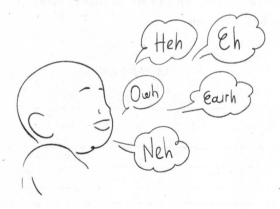

- The "HEH" sound is short, much like "NEH," so it can be confusing at times to decipher. But this sound is a clear indication that baby is uncomfortable.
- "EAIRH" sounds like a long "AIR" sound and it's usually because of digestive discomfort in the lower abdomen. Babies with colic usually make this sound. It can have a stressful piercing quality.
- The "EH" sound is a clear indication that baby has gas trapped in their upper abdomen.

Why It Works

Babies use different cries to communicate needs. The more you practice listening for the sounds and syllables of your baby's crying, the quicker you will learn to communicate with your child.

Tips

- Always check on baby if they are crying for longer than a minute or two.
- Remember, being overtired, overstimulated, or hungry are always the most likely culprits.
- If baby is crying for 3 hours or more nightly, this may be colic and your baby will benefit from a soothing daily massage.
- Record the sounds you hear in a notebook and note your remedy so you can become better at deciphering their cries over time.

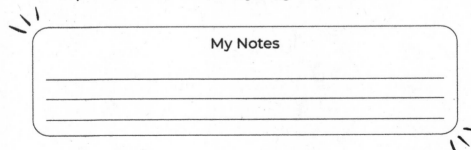

My Notes

_____

_____

_____

Hack #6

Warm It Up

Many parents wonder if warming the bottle is a necessary step, but it's a natural way to make the milk or formula easier to digest and prevents tummy upset.

Why It Works

Warm water helps formula dissolve better, thus preventing air bubbles from forming when you shake the bottle. Warming the baby's bottle, whether it's formula or breast milk, can promote deeper relaxation. Additionally, nursing at night boosts the amino acid tryptophan, which helps your baby produce more melatonin. This can lead to better sleep and gives baby a comforting sleep association.

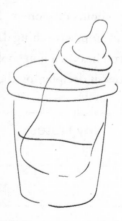

Tips

- Always test the temperature of the milk or formula before giving to baby by splashing a bit on your wrist. The milk should feel mildly warm but not hot.
- Never microwave the bottle or heat bottle directly on stove as this can lead to very hot temperatures.

How to Do It

- For stored breast milk you can either warm the milk storage bags in warm water, or pour the milk into a bottle and warm that in warm water.
- For formula, premix the bottle and warm it in a container of warm water.
- You can warm some water on the stovetop or in a bowl in the microwave at home, ask for some hot water in a large cup or bowl at a restaurant, or invest in a portable bottle warmer product like Baby's Brew.

My Notes

_____

_____

_____

_____

_____

_____

_____

Hack #7

Burping 101: The Ketchup Trick

There's no way to avoid it: Whether nursed or bottle-fed, babies will swallow air along with their milk or formula. When they are very young, it is hard for them to expel the gas on their own. If they are not burped regularly, it can result in spitting up, gassiness, and just a generally cranky baby. There are many ways to burp your baby! As you get the hang of it, you will find the best way to get that perfect, satisfying burp every time, but experiment to see what works best (and results in the least spit-up). I liked to use a method I called the Ketchup Trick.

Why It Works

When you burp your baby, you are pushing out the gas from their belly and up through the esophagus, which results in the burping sound. The Ketchup technique works well in the sitting or shoulder position because it helps to push the air up.

Tips

- Have your baby lean into your hands in the sitting position.
- Always check baby's face to see if they are struggling.
- Keep your pressure medium but not too hard.
- Have baby take frequent burp breaks during the feeding. Don't just wait to burp until the end.

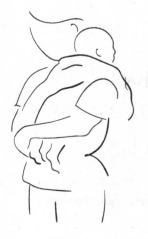 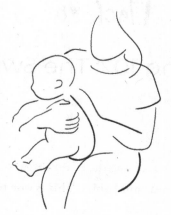 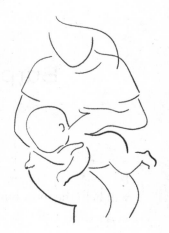

How to Do It

- Over the shoulder: Place a burp cloth on your shoulder and gently place baby's belly against your shoulder. Instead of stroking down their back or just patting their back at the top, cup your hand and stroke up from their bottom to their upper back until they burp. Lightly tap on their upper back after every four strokes or so to dislodge stubborn gas. Pat their back, but avoid hitting the spine since this area is more delicate.
- Sitting up: With baby seated on your lap, place their chin in your hand to support their head. Cup the other hand and gently pat as you stroke up from the bottom of their back in an upward motion.
- Lying down: Place your baby across your lap and gently stroke up the back, tapping on the upper back.

Hack #8

Burping 102: The Swivel

Because burping is so essential, here's a second hack that will help the most burp-resistant babies. This is one technique that helps every time.

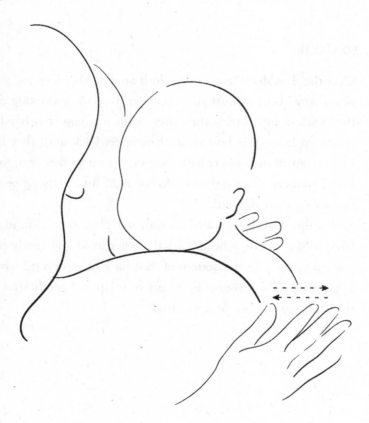

Why It Works

By swiveling the hips, you are allowing the trapped air to release and help baby either fart or burp to release the gas.

Tips

- Swivel gently at first so as not to shake baby.
- Always support their head.
- Wait 5 minutes after feeding and always have a burp cloth ready in case they spit up.

How to Do It

- Place your baby over your shoulder as if you are readying for a classic burp position.
- Instead of patting their back, use your hand to swivel their hips and bum in a figure 8 formation.
- Rub baby's back in an upward motion for ten strokes right after.
- Repeat for 1–2 minutes until baby has burped.

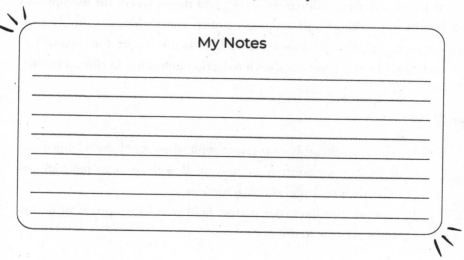

My Notes

Hack #9

Acupressure Hiccup Cure

While hiccups may seem like a mere inconvenience, some babies experience prolonged bouts of hiccups that can disrupt their schedule and peace of mind. Hiccups may be an inevitable part of life, but they don't have to interfere with your baby's well-being. The next time your wee one develops the hiccups, you can try to offer them some relief with acupressure.

Why It Works

Hiccups can erupt when the phrenic and vagus nerves are irritated, which can cause strong, involuntary rhythmic contractions of the diaphragm and intercostal muscles. Of course, babies can't be directed to hold their breath as adults and older children do to try to rid themselves of the hiccups—so besides just waiting it out, acupressure offers another way to calm the contractions. Traditional Chinese medicine calls this acupressure point BL2, and targeting this point has shown reduction in hiccups in clinical trials.

Tips

- Try massaging this acupressure point when your baby is lying down or in a Guppy position, as this can allow them to get more air and relax their neck and stomach muscles.
- You can also have your partner hold your baby upright while you apply pressure to this point.

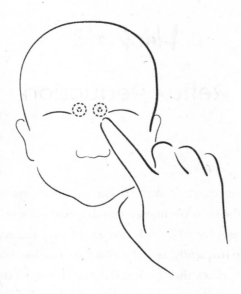

How to Do It

- Place two fingers at the point right at the start of the eyebrows, between the eyes.
- Hold with medium pressure for 10–20 seconds.
- Repeat as needed.

My Notes

_____
_____
_____
_____
_____
_____
_____
_____

Hack #10

Reflux Reduction

More than 50 percent of babies have experienced acid reflux, making it one of the most common issues that new parents face. So how do you know if your baby has it? Usually reflux babies cry and are uncomfortable after eating, hiccup frequently, arch their back after eating, and hate being flat on their back. Also, check their breath. If it smells sour, it's definitely reflux.

There are many ways to manage reflux, and most babies will outgrow it by the time they are 12 months old. While some doctors will want to prescribe medicine, you can try natural holistic techniques first. Baby massage can help!

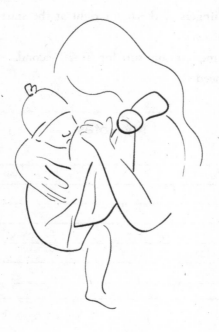

Why It Works

A full-body massage can help with the vagus nerve function. This nerve (actually a system of multiple cranial nerves) extends from the brain to the large intestine and regulates digestion, among many other involuntary body functions. Baby massage helps to accelerate nerve maturation, helping your baby's nerves develop faster and operate most efficiently to help control the muscle between the esophagus and the stomach.

Tips

- Keep your baby upright as long as possible (20–30 minutes) or in an elevated position after feeding. You can use a baby carrier or a jumper type of product once they reach 6 months.
- Try a natural remedy like Natrum Phosphoricum, known as Nat Pho. It replaces the natural levels of cell salt our bodies need for optimal digestion.

How to Do It

- Refer to the Basic Baby Massage section on page 14 for directions.

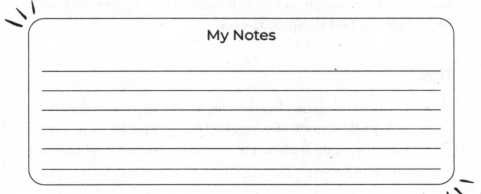

My Notes

_____
_____
_____
_____
_____
_____

Hack #11

No "Fast Food" for Reflux

Slow it down! You may not be aware that the pace that you are feeding your baby may cause gassiness and reflux. Slowing down bottle-feeding with a practice called paced feeding can help babies suffering from reflux and other digestive issues. (Note: Nursing moms can try pressing a hand into the side of the breast during letdown to slow down the flow of milk.)

Why It Works

When baby swallows the milk or formula, it goes through the lower esophageal sphincter (LES) to the stomach. In reflux babies, the LES muscles don't close and open on cue, and food can come back through the esophagus, leading to vomiting, spit-up, and general fussiness and discomfort. By keeping your baby upright as long as possible and taking frequent breaks, you will give the food more time to settle.

Tips

- Use a foam wedge or place them higher on your chest while feeding.
- If they fall asleep after feeding, hold baby upright for a few minutes before laying them down. For safe sleep, never place any reclining objects in the crib.

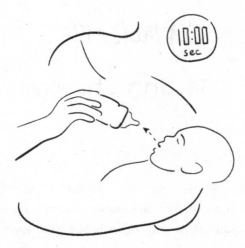

How to Do It

- Try feeding your baby in an upright position rather than lying down flat.
- Hold the bottle horizontally rather than tilted down into baby's mouth.
- Let baby take three to five swallows (about 20–30 seconds).
- To give baby a break, tip the base of the bottle toward the floor so that the milk or formula isn't filling the nipple.
- When baby starts to suck again, level the bottle to let milk or formula back into the nipple.
- Repeat until baby shows signs of being full and satisfied, then end the feeding.

Hack #12

Getting Cheeky

Many parents assume that babies are just natural milk or formula guzzlers and can feed on command (I was no exception!). And while many *are* quite adept at it, other babies need special oral exercises and warm-up massages to help them become more efficient feeders. This massage helps to support a baby's oral motor development.

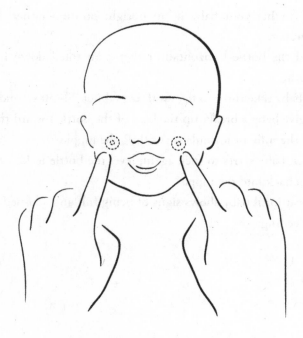

Why It Works

This facial massage strengthens oral musculature and promotes jaw mobility so baby can be a more effective nurser and can improve the efficiency of their sucking mechanism, drawing out more milk.

Tips

- Try this technique if you see baby is not feeding enough or not latching properly.
- Repeat a few times a day but make sure to pause if baby seems uncomfortable. You can try again in 20 minutes or wait until after their next nap.
- Massage gently but with enough pressure to help your baby develop better muscle tone.

How to Do It

- Use your index and middle finger and draw small circles starting at baby's ears down their cheeks to the chin.
- Press gently into baby's cheeks, making sure baby is comfortable.
- Repeat on the other side of baby's face.
- Massage baby's lips.

My Notes

_____
_____
_____
_____

Hack #13

Tongue of War

Tongue exercises are a great way to build strength and expand your baby's oral motor range, giving them a head start on feeding and helping them develop a strong latch.

Why It Works

This technique helps to strengthen the tongue muscles and develop oral motor strength. By pretending to tug and remove your finger, you are encouraging baby to suck and move the tongue forward.

Tips

- Always trim your nails and wash your hands before starting.
- Your baby's mouth could be very sensitive. Work on this technique slowly and don't pull too hard. You can increase the suction once your baby gets more used to it.
- Do this exercise three times every day.

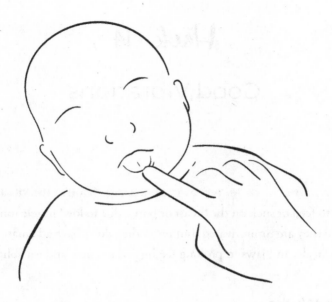

How to Do It

- Wash your hands thoroughly.
- Stroke your baby's lower lip and allow them to suck your index finger into their mouth.
- Gently pull your finger away, creating a tug-of-war effect where baby tries to draw your finger into their mouth.
- Repeat the sequence three or four times.

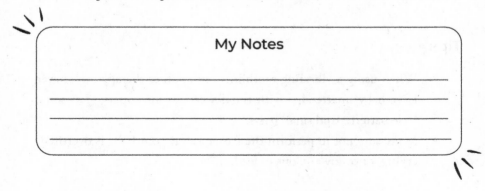

My Notes

Hack #14

Good Vibrations

Some babies have a hard time using their jaw and cheek muscles to feed or suck on the breast or bottle due to low muscle tone. It may seem like they are unmotivated, but often they don't have adequate strength in their cheeks and jaws to prolong feeding or to chew and eat solids.

Why It Works

Vibration is used by physical and occupational therapists to help build oral motor strength and improve everything from feeding to speech impediments. The gentle vibration provides tactile sensory input that helps babies and tots become more aware of their mouth, tongue, and jaw muscles, bringing more attention to that area so they can learn to use their muscles more efficiently. Sometimes babies can get sleepy and these facial stimulation exercises can wake them up and stimulate their facial muscles so they are more productive feeders.

Tips

- When using a vibrating toothbrush or another therapy tool, never leave baby unattended with the device. Always supervise as some have batteries and small parts.
- Make sure not to perform these exercises if your baby is overtired, crying, or overly anxious to feed.

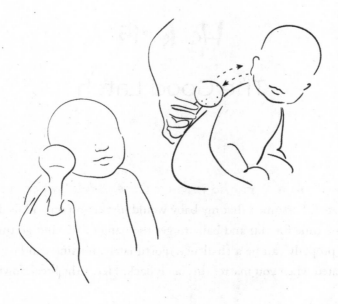

How to Do It

- Use a gentle vibrating instrument to massage baby's face. You can use a vibrating toothbrush or the Kahlmi massage wand to massage their cheeks along the jawline to create a sensation that helps to wake up your baby's facial muscles.
- Place the vibrating object on your baby's tongue to help draw awareness to this area and encourage a stronger sucking motion.
- Repeat these exercises before feeding three times a day for 5 minutes each time to achieve desired tone and facial muscle awareness.

My Notes

Hack #15

The Good Latch

As a new mom, I had no idea that breastfeeding could be so complicated. I assumed that my baby would just clamp on and feed. It can take some time for you and baby to get the hang of it—and getting them to latch properly can be a challenge. Fortunately, nursing can be a lot less complicated when you master this latch hack. Here's the breakdown.

Why It Works

When baby doesn't latch properly and just latches to the tip of the nipple, you will experience more pain and your baby will have a harder time nursing. Also, by touching their face with your nipple prior to latching, it helps to stimulate your baby's natural rooting reflex.

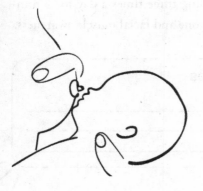
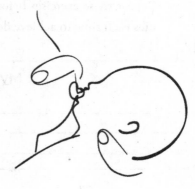

Tips

- Make sure your baby's chin is touching your breast.
- Check if baby's tongue is wrapped around the breast in a cup formation.
- If the latch is hurting your nipple, insert your finger to break the seal and start again.

 ## How to Do It

- Place your baby so that their stomach is touching yours and make sure you are supporting their head and body with your arm and a pillow.
- Position their chin at the bottom of the nipple and wait till they open their mouth wide to insert the nipple.
- Once they have latched, use your finger to move the bottom lip down and away from the nipple to widen their mouth further.
- Make sure your baby has engulfed the entire nipple in their mouth and their lips are splayed outward rather than puckered in.

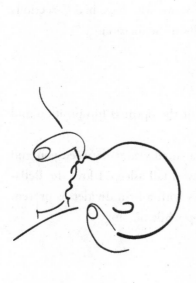

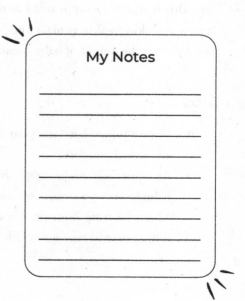

My Notes

Hack #16

Side Sleeper Nursing Position

Many nursing moms default to the sitting-up position, but one of the most natural and effective ways of nursing is the side-lying position. Not only does it allow mom to rest and be more comfortable, it's also a great way to get skin to skin with baby since their stomach is right next to yours. If feeding at night, prevent yourself from falling asleep or rolling over by placing a small pillow wedge between you and baby to ensure a safety barrier.

Why It Works

The side-lying position allows you and baby to fully relax and ease into nursing. This is widely recommended as the best position for new moms since it increases skin-to-skin contact and helps moms who have had C-sections recover since the weight of baby doesn't fall on the incision.

Tips

- Place a pillow between your legs for the optimal hip position and additional comfort.
- At night or if you're sleepy, place a small wedge between you and baby so that you can't roll over if you fall asleep. I love the Bella-Moon Nursing Nest since it comes with a firm divider to prevent rolling over in case mom falls asleep while nursing.

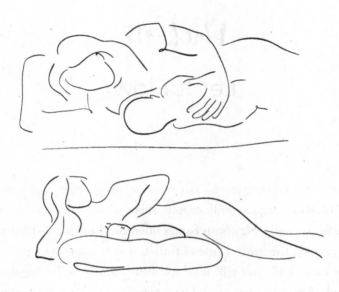

How to Do It

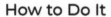

- Lie down with one arm supporting your head.
- Position baby against your body. Make sure your baby's mouth is lined up with your breast, and use your free arm to draw them to you.
- Support your back with a pillow while baby nurses.
- When one breast has been emptied, repeat the process on the other side. You can roll over if you need to, but you may be able to simply adjust your angle to offer baby access to the other breast.

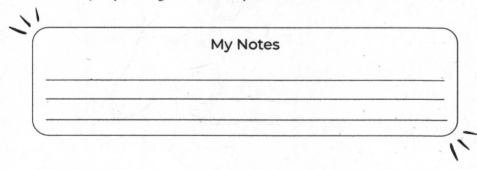

My Notes

_____

_____

_____

Hack #17

Let It Flow

One of the biggest hurdles for moms who want to breastfeed is establishing an adequate milk supply. There are so many ways to increase milk supply naturally. Newborn babies often need to feed 8–12 times in a 24-hour period. The general rule of thumb is that the more you feed your baby, the more milk you will produce. But if you're still struggling with milk supply, here are some natural hacks that can increase your supply.

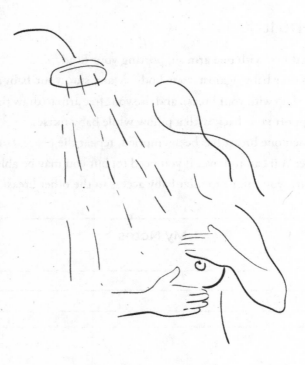

Why It Works

Massaging your breasts and your baby releases oxytocin in both of you, which helps with milk flow. By pumping and feeding your baby often, your body also produces more milk. The more you feed on demand, the higher your supply will be.

Tips

- When it comes to milk production, it's very common for mothers to worry about providing an adequate supply. As long as your baby is gaining weight and thriving, try to give yourself grace and understand that every mother produces a different amount of milk.
- Try to relax before and during a feeding session. Spend time massaging your neck and breast area as well as your baby so you can ease into the nursing session and produce more milk.
- I love the brand Legendairy Milk for their herbal supplements, which have a devoted following among moms.

How to Do It

- Take a hot shower before you feed baby and massage your breasts in the shower.
- Use a vibrating tool like a lactation massager while you feed baby to help with letdown.
- Pump for 15 minutes after feeding (both breasts).
- Manually massage your breast while baby is nursing.
- Massage your baby during the nursing session.

Hack #18

Pain Points

Whoever tells you that nursing won't hurt in the beginning is telling a white lie or suffering from amnesia. It's not easy at first, and the discomfort *will* go away. Here's a hack to help alleviate and manage pain in the early stages so you can continue relatively pain free on your breastfeeding journey. (Or not! Because as the saying goes, fed is best.)

Why It Works

Coconut and olive oil have natural anti-inflammatory properties and can heal dry, cracked skin naturally. In a 2015 study, researchers found that olive oil actually treated and prevented cracking with no adverse side effects.

Tips

- While they are not recommended for long-term use, nipple shields can be a lifesaver in the beginning while your skin gets acclimated to nursing.
- When it comes to boobs, women know one size does NOT fit all. If you're pumping, the pump parts might be the issue. Standard pumps come with parts that are designed for only a few sizes. For best results, it's important to measure oneself to find the right flange size and also try cushion inserts from companies like BeauGen to minimize nipple pain.

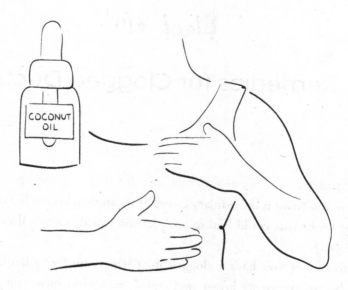

Things to Try

- Coconut and/or olive oil is amazing to apply on nipples and works better to reduce nipple cracking and pain than over-the-counter ointments. Apply a small amount to each nipple day and night, as needed.
- While you will want to wipe the oil off your breast before nursing, it is all natural and nontoxic to baby, so if small amounts get in their mouth it won't harm them.
- Let the oil absorb into your skin overnight.

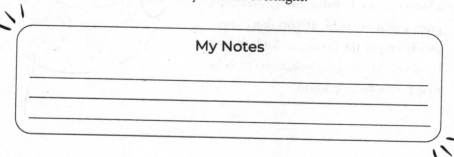

My Notes

Hack #19

Remedies for Clogged Ducts

Clogged milk ducts are a big issue for nursing moms. Trapped milk in the breast is the primary cause. This can then lead to inflammation in the breast that could lead to an infection called mastitis if not treated right away.

You know you have a clogged duct when you feel a hard lump in your breast, experience breast swelling, or see a white blister on your nipple. While antibiotics are the standard treatment for mastitis, there are natural ways to help heal and stave off clogged milk ducts before they turn into a full-fledged infection.

Why It Works

Blocked milk ducts can be caused by a variety of reasons, such as poor latch or a longer period between feeds, like dropping a feed at night. If you don't completely empty the breast, it can lead to a blockage. Massaging the breasts can help to get milk flowing again.

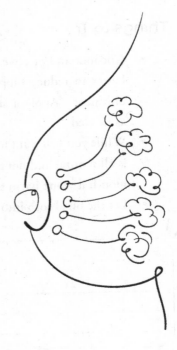

Tips

- Try to pump a little extra after every feed. Not only will you collect more milk, it will help empty the breasts.
- Massage and place heat on your breast during every nursing session.
- If you don't have a massager, use your hands to massage your breasts.

Things to Try

- Cabbage leaves may seem like an old superstition, but it's amazing what it can do to relieve pain in the breast. Wash cabbage leaves and pat them dry with a paper towel. Tuck a leaf into your bra and wear until it is wilted. Continue to replace the leaf until the engorgement has subsided. Note: Use this trick sparingly as cabbage leaves can decrease milk supply.
- Fill a Haakaa breast pump with warm water and 1–2 tablespoons of Epsom salt and attach to the affected breast. Keep on for 10–15 minutes and repeat as necessary.
- While recent guidance from the Academy of Breastfeeding Medicine urges caution around the use of massage and vibration as they can promote rather than reduce inflammation, many moms swear by them to loosen plugs. Place a warm towel on your breast and use a Kahlmi massager or a lactation massager to massage the breast for 1–3 minutes.
- Always try to empty the affected breast as much as possible with frequent nursing sessions and pumping after feeding your baby.
- To combat occasional inflammation of the breasts, apply heat and massage the breast before nursing or pumping, and follow nursing or pumping sessions with cold compresses.

Hack #20

Eyes on the Prize

As your baby gets older, their senses become sharper and more developed, which is wonderful and important. Yet with this developmental growth, distracted feeding can become an issue and may prevent your baby from focusing on the nursing task at hand and emptying the breasts efficiently.

One good hack for keeping your baby focused while you nurse is to wear a nursing necklace so your baby can pull on it and play with it rather than twisting their head to get a look around the room.

Why It Works

A silicone edible-grade necklace is a great way to keep your baby from nipping, turning their head, and being distracted by all the sights and sounds around them.

Tips

- Use an edible-grade silicone necklace as this can be repurposed for teething later on.
- Introduce your baby to the necklace for a few minutes prior to nursing so it can be viewed as something rare and desirable.
- Never leave your baby unattended with the necklace on their own.
- Try to nurse in a quiet, dim room.

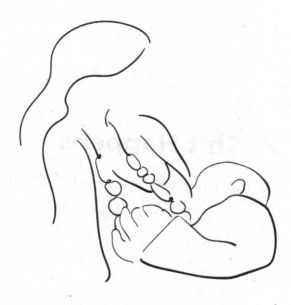

How to Do It

- Choose a necklace with high-contrast silicone beads that are safe for baby.
- Only wear the necklace when you are nursing so that your baby gets excited by the newness of the toy.
- A necklace also serves as a nursing cue, helping your baby understand it's time to feed.

My Notes

_____

_____

_____

_____

_____

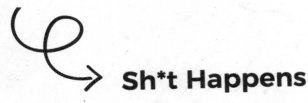

Sh*t Happens

17 Hacks for Gas, Constipation, and Diarrhea

There is one topic every couple will spend hours dissecting and discussing in far more detail than they could ever imagine: poop! Few parents expect their lives to be completely upended to revolve around going number two. But it's a huge issue for babies. Babies are born with immature digestive systems, which means their bowels don't work optimally until at least 3–4 months. They spit up frequently, suffer from gas pain, and poop or don't poop at the most inopportune times. This means you'll need to give your baby a helping hand in moving the milk or formula around to decrease blockages, release gas, and get everything back on track. While many of these symptoms go away after 4 months or so, it's hard on both baby and parents so make sure you give yourself plenty of support and grace.

Poop and gas can stymie parents because there is so much variation from baby to baby. What's normal for one isn't necessarily normal for another. And what's normal for your baby today may be entirely different tomorrow. In the newborn days, babies will poop a lot. As they get older, the range for what's normal can be all over the place, with some babies pooping three times a day and others pooping just once a week.

Breastfed babies and formula-fed babies are also quite different in their pooping styles and schedules because breast milk and formula are digested differently. Breastfed babies will often not need to poop for several days, while formula-fed babies tend to poop at least daily. If they are gaining weight steadily and passing stool without much issue, everything is fine.

About 30 percent of children will deal with constipation at some point. Constipation usually happens when the colon absorbs too much water and dries out baby's stool. This causes their poop to be harder, which can prevent elimination and slow down the bowel transit time. Watch your child for signs of straining when they're trying to poop, a swollen belly, or hard, pebble-like stool.

Babies can also suffer from gas buildup and the dreaded colic, which is unexplained crying lasting over 3 hours. While many doctors still don't know the exact cause of colic, many believe it has to do with the gut, gas, and immature digestion.

Research clearly shows that baby massage can help with symptoms of all types of digestive issues. One study found that infant massage helps to stimulate the vagus nerve, a nerve that carries signals between the brain, heart, and digestive system. Yet another study found that infant massage increases defecation frequency and reduces constipation in babies with chronic issues. There are many different methods that parents try to help relieve their baby of any troubling digestive issues. However, baby massage is the most effective method to help relieve constipation and baby gas.

So when in doubt and when it feels like your baby will never get over their digestive issues, try out these massage strokes and natural hacks. (If your baby continues to struggle even after trying out all these natural techniques, make sure to consult your pediatrician.)

Hack #1

I Love You

A regular tummy massage is essential to keeping your baby's digestive system operating at optimal levels. Sometimes babies will experience gas and bloating, which can be remedied easily and quickly with a daily belly massage. The I Love You massage is one my favorites since it's easy to learn. For this stroke, you will be tracing the letters *I*, *L*, and *U* (for "I love you") on your baby's body.

Why It Works

ILU massage helps stimulate abdominal muscle contractions and facilitates easier bowel movements.

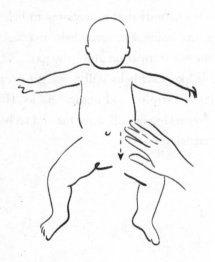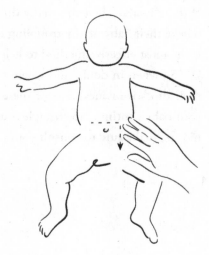

Tip

- Perform the belly strokes two to three times daily for optimal results.

How to Do It

- Start on the left side of your baby's belly and use the tips of your fingers to trace an *I*, starting right under their rib and ending right above the pubic bone.
- Move your hand to the right side of your baby's belly and trace an upside-down *L* on your baby's tummy. Start on the far side of the right rib and work toward the center of your baby's belly. When you reach the center, go straight down toward their belly button.
- Trace an upside-down *U* on your baby's belly. Start near baby's right hip, and move your fingers in a curve that goes up to their sternum and then back down toward the opposite hip.
- Use medium pressure as if you are kneading dough.
- Repeat the *I-L-U* sequence ten times.

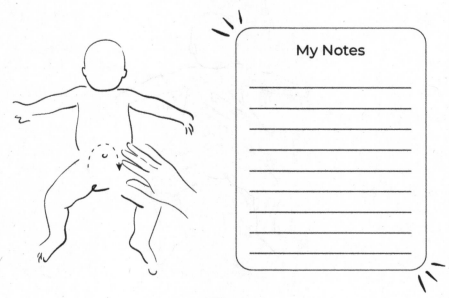

My Notes

Hack #2

Sun and Moon

The sun and moon belly massage is a gentle but medium-
pressure tummy massage that can help the digestive tract work optimally.
It's easy to do whenever you're changing your baby or during a bath or just
lounging around the house.

Why It Works

The massage follows the direction of the digestive tract, helping to reduce
gas bubbles and calm your baby. It allows you to move gas through the
intestinal tract and toward the bowels.

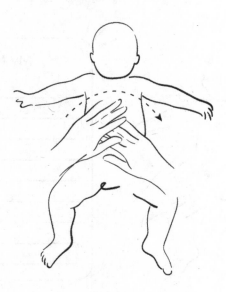

Tips

- Never massage your baby's belly right after feeding. Wait at least 20–30 minutes.
- Make sure one hand stays in contact with baby at all times to create a sense of security.
- Use a massage oil to create a gentle gliding motion.

How to Do It

- Use your hands to make clockwise circles on baby's belly with medium pressure. (Always follow the digestive tract and move clockwise on your baby's right side to their left.)
- Go slow and alternate between hands so that one hand always maintains contact with baby's body.
- Repeat this stroke for 3–5 minutes.

My Notes

_____
_____
_____
_____
_____
_____
_____
_____

Hack #3

Fulling

This stroke helps eliminate gas and air that may be stuck in the upper digestive tract.

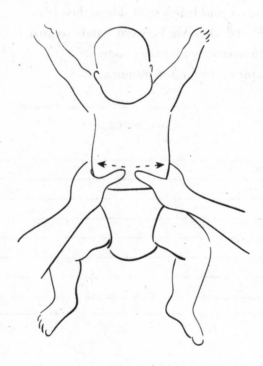

Why It Works

The fulling stroke follows the direction of the digestive tract, helping to reduce gas bubbles and calm baby. Studies suggest that baby massage can stimulate the vagus nerve, leading to better digestion and improved absorption of vital nutrients.

Tips

- Use a flat thumb so as not to poke baby.
- Do not make contact with the belly button.

How to Do It

- Place your two thumbs flat on baby's belly.
- Using medium pressure, press in on the belly while sliding your thumbs outward to the sides of baby's body.
- Repeat this same motion as you work your way from the top of the belly down to the pelvis. Do two strokes above the belly button, two strokes at the level of the belly button, and two strokes beneath the belly button.

My Notes

_____
_____
_____
_____
_____
_____
_____

Hack #4

Paddling

Paddling is another great belly massage stroke to help move trapped air and can help your baby with colic or other gastrointestinal issues.

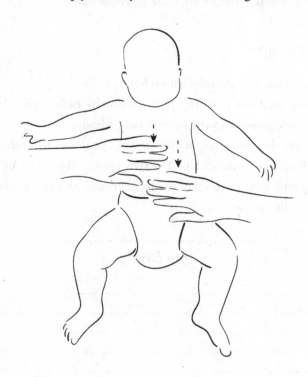

Why It Works

Baby massage strokes that target the belly help to tone the gastrointestinal tract and to relieve gas and constipation.

Tips

- Always wait 20–30 minutes after feeding to massage baby's belly.
- Warm your hands before placing them on your baby's belly by rubbing them together.
- Use a drop of edible-grade organic oil like coconut or jojoba oil when massaging baby's tummy.

How to Do It

- Close up all your fingers to form two paddles with your hands.
- Using the side of one closed paddle hand, stroke from your baby's upper rib cage to their pelvis.
- Alternate hands so that you maintain constant contact with baby's belly.
- Always stroke in a downward direction.

My Notes

_____
_____
_____
_____
_____
_____
_____

Hack #5

Dire Straits

Diarrhea is a normal part of baby life. While you should not be alarmed by occasional diarrhea, it is important to properly treat your baby if symptoms occur. Frequent watery poops are the main indicators of diarrhea, which can be caused by viral infection, food allergies, and medication (especially antibiotics). The most important rule is to keep your baby hydrated. Here are a few massage tricks that will help your baby.

Why It Works

Counterclockwise belly massage slows the frequency and intensity of loose bowel movements and can significantly decrease diarrhea.

Tips

- Watch out for signs of dehydration, such as lethargy, decrease in urine, or diarrhea that lasts more than a few days.
- If your baby has started on solids, try feeding them mashed bananas or rice cereal as a natural diarrhea deterrent. If the diarrhea is triggered by antibiotics, and your baby is 4–6 months or older, try feeding your baby some no-sugar-added yogurt, which is full of helpful probiotics.

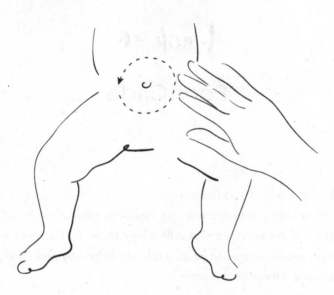

How to Do It

- Using the pad of your hand, massage baby's belly counterclockwise, starting from left to right.
- Repeat for 3–5 minutes, three times a day until symptoms improve.

My Notes

_____
_____
_____
_____
_____
_____
_____

Hack #6

Foot Glide

Reflexology for your baby's feet is an incredible way to help you ease your baby's constipation and gassiness. One of my most popular videos on social media is the foot reflexology massage. Parents are amazed that a simple foot massage can be all it takes to help baby poop and get their bowels moving. Here's how to start.

Why It Works

Foot reflexology is an Eastern therapy that applies pressure to specific points on the feet. The practice is based on the idea that there are reflex zones on the feet that correspond to various organs and that pressing on one of these points can relieve blockages in that part of the body. These two lines correspond to the intestines and are known to release blockage there.

Tips

- Pressure is very important here. Be sure to use medium pressure. Too hard, and baby will not enjoy it. But if too light, baby will get ticklish.
- To ground them and warm up baby's foot, hold your palm against the sole of your baby's foot.

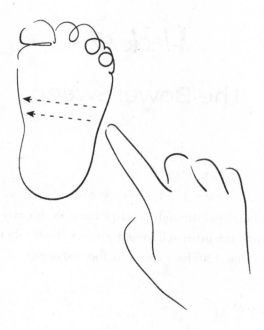

How to Do It

- Use your index finger and stroke the two lines shown here, using medium pressure.
- The top line, located right below the fleshy pad of baby's foot, corresponds to the small intestine.
- The bottom line, located just above the heel, corresponds to the large intestine.
- Stroke from the outside of the foot to the inside on both feet.

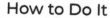

My Notes

_____

_____

_____

Hack #7

The Bowel Sweep

When baby is constipated, this stroke really works well to move the flow of material through the large intestine. It's easy to do and can be combined with the other reflexology strokes (Foot Glide on page 116 and Fanning on page 120) for a complete foot massage.

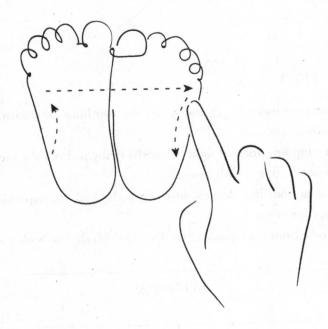

Why It Works

This stroke helps to stimulate the large intestine, promoting movement of the bowels.

Tips

- Use an organic massage oil to help your fingers glide.
- If your baby pulls their feet away or cries, stop and try again later.

How to Do It

- Using your thumb or index finger, slide your finger up the outer side of the left foot and draw across, using medium pressure.
- Continue the movement on the other foot, moving across to the outside edge of the right foot and going down.
- Repeat this stroke from left to right five to ten times.

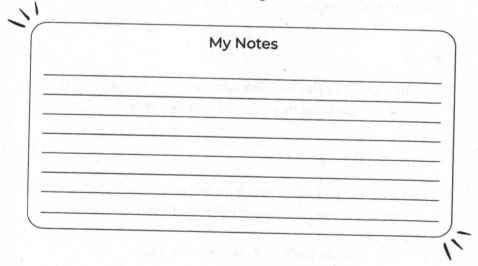

My Notes

Hack #8

Fanning

This is a nice way to get your baby's foot warmed up. Sometimes your baby can be a little squeamish if you start reflexology right away and fanning helps prepare your baby's foot for deeper reflexology stimulation.

Why It Works

This massage stroke provides pressure to the entire foot, helping to prepare your baby's foot for deeper massage and getting them used to the sensation of having their feet touched.

Tip

- Be mindful of pressure. Too light, and your baby might feel ticklish. Too hard, and they may pull their foot away.

How to Do It

- Using your thumbs, stroke up the sole of your baby's foot from the heel to the toes, one thumb following the other. Apply medium pressure.
- Move up to the pad directly beneath baby's toes.
- Repeat three to five times, then switch to the other foot.

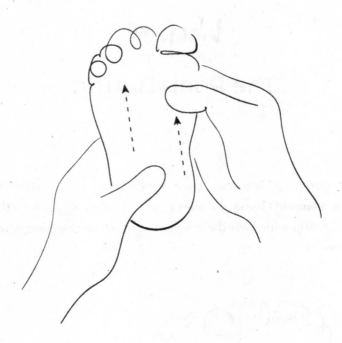

My Notes

_____
_____
_____
_____
_____
_____
_____
_____
_____

Hack #9

The Poop Button

Did you know your baby has a "poop button" on their body? Yes, a poop button! One of the most powerful reflexology points, the solar plexus, can help with even the toughest bouts of constipation when activated properly.

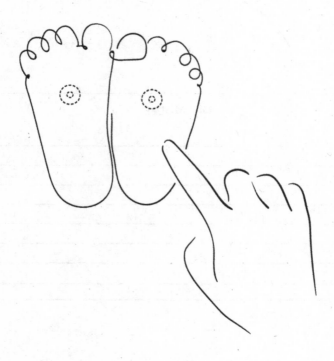

Why It Works

The solar plexus has been called the abdominal nerve center and is considered in traditional Chinese medicine to be one of the most important areas of the body's energy system.

Tips

- Always massage this area on both feet to balance the body.
- The solar plexus is a very powerful point so check on your baby to make sure the pressure is right for them. Signs they are uncomfortable include fussing, arching their back, and pulling their feet away.
- A little oil can help you massage this area and will be super relaxing for your baby, releasing tension and leading to easier bowel movements.

How to Do It

- The solar plexus is activated by pressing the slight indentation right below the ball of the foot and in line between the second and third toes.
- Use your thumbs to press on this area on both feet for 1 minute with medium pressure.
- Make small circles in a clockwise motion on both feet, using a deeper pressure for 2 minutes.

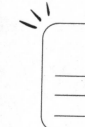

My Notes

_____

_____

_____

Hack #10

Stomach Jiu-Jitsu

There is one point on your baby's leg/shin that really helps regulate their digestion, constipation, gas pains, and even diarrhea. It's as easy as applying pressure to this spot for 1–2 minutes on both sides of the shins.

Why It Works

Known as the Stomach 36, Zusanli, or Leg Three Mile Point, massaging this point helps with all things related to baby's digestion, including gas, tummy pains, nausea, and constipation.

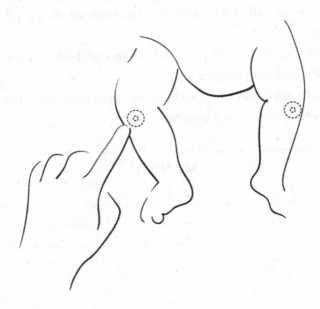

Tip

- Watch your baby carefully to see how they react. Pause the massage if you notice signs of discomfort, which include fussiness, crying, and tensing muscles.

How to Do It

- Locate this point by sliding your fingers down baby's knee about the width of two to three fingers on the baby's shin.
- Use medium pressure and hold the point for 30 seconds. Then, make small circles here for another 30 seconds.
- Repeat on the other shin. Do this massage two to three times a day.

My Notes

Hack #11

Palm-Aid

The hands, like the feet and ears, have many reflexology points to help clear energy blockages in the body. This reflexology hack activates a point associated with better digestion.

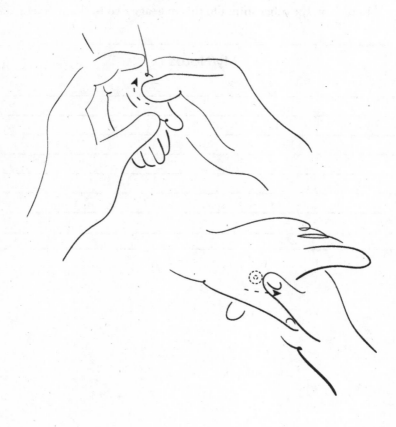

Why It Works

According to Chinese reflexology, the hands contain many nerve endings. When pressure is applied, these pathways are energized. The L14 point on the hand helps with digestion, reflux, and other gastrointestinal difficulties.

Tip

- You can use your thumb to make small circular motions, knead the area between baby's fingers and thumb, or use your fingers to apply a gentle squeezing motion. Experiment with different techniques to find what feels most effective and comfortable for your baby.

How to Do It

- Warm up baby's palms by making brisk circles on the inside of their palms with your thumbs, using medium pressure.
- Locate the fleshy webbing between baby's thumb and index finger on one hand.
- Pinch here gently using light pressure. Start with gentle pressure and slowly increase to medium or even to firm pressure based on your baby's reactions.
- Make small kneading circles on this area for 1–2 minutes.
- Repeat on the other hand.

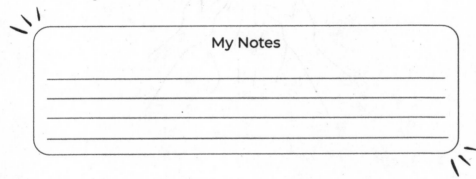

My Notes

Hack #12

Figure 8

While there are many bodywork massage techniques to help stimulate digestion and elimination, this one is a personal favorite since it helps exercise the hips and relax their spine as well.

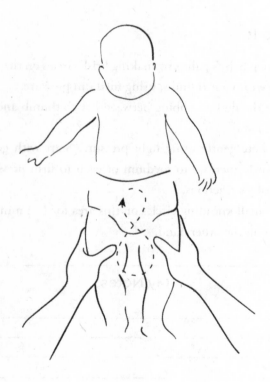

Why It Works

While bicycle kicks and tummy circles work for many babies, other babies will need this additional bodywork to create more space for the milk to flow through.

Tip

- Always watch your baby's reaction so you never push and sway their hips beyond their comfort zone.

How to Do It

- Roll your baby onto their back and place your thumbs on baby's abdomen. Wrap your hands around baby's hips, with your thumbs securely at the top of their hips.
- Move baby's entire pelvic region in a clockwise direction. Repeat for 1 minute.
- Move baby's hips in a figure 8 formation for about 2 minutes.
- Repeat the entire sequence again for 2 minutes.

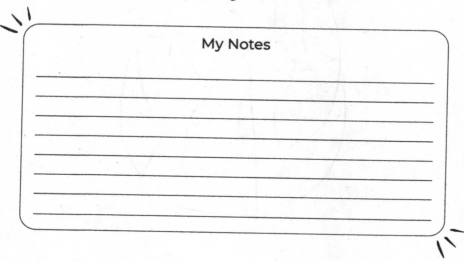

My Notes

Hack #13

The Trifecta: Bath, Tummy Massage, Bicycles

There are times you will have to bring out the big guns and combine a few hacks to deal with stubborn constipation. Here's a one-two-three punch that not even the most stubborn poop can resist.

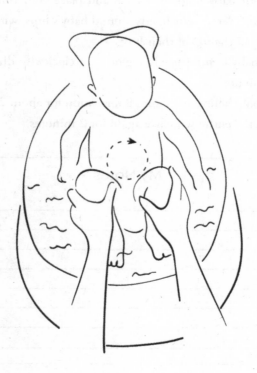

Why It Works

Warm water helps to stimulate blood flow and circulation, which promotes bowel movements. It also relieves body tension, allowing your baby to relax their gastrointestinal tract. Following up with belly massage and leg bicycling takes advantage of that relaxation to get everything moving again.

Tips

- Use a smaller baby bathtub so if baby poops it is contained and can be easily cleaned.
- Set a relaxing mood for the bath scene. Dim the lights so baby can fully relax. A relaxed baby is able to eliminate stool more easily.

How to Do It

- Start with a warm bath. Let your baby soak. While they are in the bath, gently lift baby so you can access their bottom. Use a small towel to energize their anus, rubbing gently to stimulate. When bath time is done, dry baby thoroughly with a towel.
- Massage baby's belly using clockwise circles and other techniques outlined in this chapter.
- Finish by stretching their legs straight, pulling gently, followed by bicycle movements to help move the poop around.

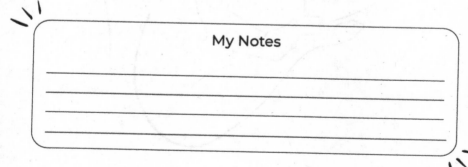

My Notes

_____

_____

_____

_____

Hack #14

Toilet Position

Let's face it. Pooping while lying down is not the ideal position. As adults, we have the benefit of sitting up on the toilet to do our business. Babies who can't sit up by themselves have a hard time getting into an optimal potty position. When it's been days and baby hasn't shown any signs of poop, it's time to help them along with this body positioning hack.

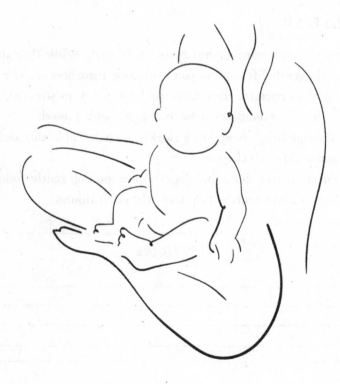

Why It Works

Ever tried pooping while lying down? Not so easy. This is the correct anatomical position for optimal poop that will help your baby get the stool out.

Tips

- Try bouncing your baby on your legs a bit to get things moving.
- Make sure your baby's knees are pushed up a little toward their belly to maximize the impact.

How to Do It

- Sit in a comfortable cross-legged position on the floor.
- Place your baby in the middle of the hole created by the crossing of your legs.
- Let their legs fall over your legs.
- Hold this position for 5–10 minutes while letting your baby play with toys or reading them a book.

My Notes

_____
_____
_____
_____
_____
_____
_____
_____

Hack #15

1-2-3 Squat

Using different positions to help your baby poop is a great way to troubleshoot when they are backed up. It's easy to do, provided you make sure baby has plenty of head support.

Why It Works

By holding your baby in a squatting position, the body is in a more natural position for optimal pooping. The squatting position straightens the rectum and relaxes the rectal muscles, helping to clear the path.

Tips

- You can hold this position on a stable surface. Or, for smaller babies, support them against your chest while drawing their knees up.
- For older babies, try tandem sitting on the toilet seat. Sit far back on the seat, with your legs open over the toilet bowl. Place your hands under baby's knees to make a "seat" with your hands and let them lean back against you. This will also encourage earlier potty training and positive associations with the toilet bowl. You'll be surprised how important this is later on when the toilet bowl becomes their mortal enemy.

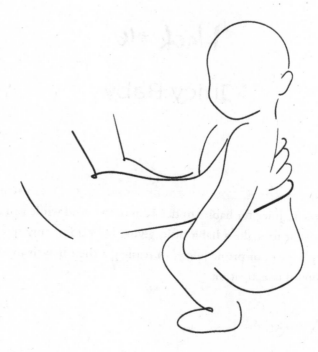

How to Do It

- Hold your baby right under their armpits.
- Let their feet gently touch the floor or any stable surface.
- Help them get into a squatting position by letting their bottom sink a little deeper and their knees bend as you hold them upright. Hold for 20–30 seconds and repeat two to three times at different times of the day until the baby has successfully passed stool.

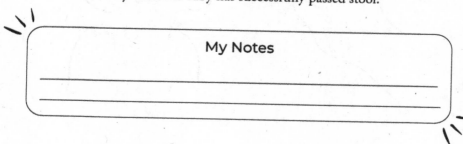

My Notes

_____

_____

Hack #16

Juicy Baby

We know. We know. The American Academy of Pediatrics does not recommend juice for babies under 12 months. And while you certainly would not want to make a habit of it, giving baby a few tiny spoonfuls of organic apple, pear, or prune juice can really get their bowels moving after a longer bout of constipation.

Why It Works

Prunes, apples, and pears contain natural fibers that can add bulk to the stool and help to stimulate bowel movements.

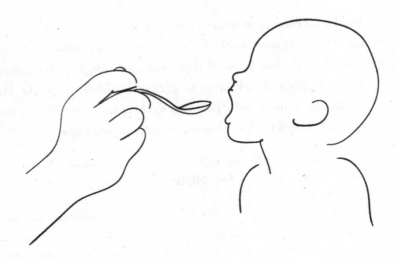

Tips

- Always opt for homemade juice using organic fruit rather than store-bought juices, which have a lot of sugar (even no-sugar-added varieties).
- Limit offering juice to once a day, and only increase the dose if the previous amount was ineffectual.
- Make sure to thoroughly cool the juice before giving it to baby.

How to Do It

- Boil an organic apple, pear, or prune in a small pot of water until soft.
- Place the boiled fruit into a blender with 2 tablespoons of water reserved from the pot. Blend until smooth.
- Take 2 tablespoons of fruit puree and mix with ⅓ cup boiled water to make juice.
- Cool the mixture.
- Give baby 2–4 ounces using a spoon.
- Store extra juice in a glass container in the fridge for 2–3 days, or freeze it in a BPA-free ice tray for up to 30 days. To serve, warm the juice to thaw, and let it cool to room temperature before feeding it to your baby.

My Notes

_____
_____
_____
_____
_____

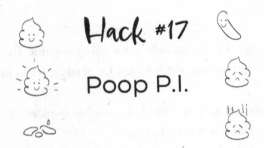

Hack #17
Poop P.I.

Every new parent at some point will find themselves with the unusual task of investigating and inspecting their baby's poop. You won't believe how adept you will become at decoding your baby's poop by the time they are 3 months old. Your pediatrician may even occasionally ask you to take some photos of your baby's poop to see if there is cause for alarm or need for a doctor's visit. I can't tell you how many times we had to take photos and send them around to members of the extended family to get poop consensus. Here's a quick guide to deciphering your baby's poop.

Why It Works

Your baby's poop is an indicator of a healthy microbiome, which is a group of microbes that impact their immunity and nutrient absorption. Learning to be a poop detective is a time-tested tradition all parents will go through and it can help you understand how your baby's primary systems are functioning.

Tips

- Don't panic if your baby's poop seems off. There are a lot of variations on what is normal.
- Always get a second opinion from your doctor if your baby's poop falls into one of the two concerning categories.
- Take your baby to the doctor right away if their poop falls into the third category.

Normal Poop

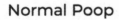

- Yellow and seedy: Breastfed babies have loose, yellow, seedy poop with a mild smell. It may look like diarrhea, but it is completely normal for babies who are exclusively breastfed to have poop of this consistency.
- Dark and thick: Formula-fed babies will usually have a darker poop color. The texture is often thick.
- Green and brown/black: A new baby's stools (also called meconium) are usually dark and appear greenish-black. This is perfectly normal. This color can also appear if baby is starting on solids or if your child is taking iron supplements.

Second Opinion

- Watery and runny: This can be a sign of diarrhea, so watch your baby carefully. If this continues for more than 2 days, you will want to talk to your doctor.
- Dry and pebbly: This is a sign of constipation. To remedy, try some of the hacks in this chapter.
- Greenish and slimy: This can indicate mucus in poop and can be a sign of an infection; consult with your pediatrician.
- Very smelly: While some smells are perfectly normal, if you detect an unusually strong scent, check with your baby's doctor.

Red Alert (Immediate visit to the doctor)

- Whitish or chalky poop: This is a sign that your baby is producing bile, a digestive fluid made in the liver. It signals that they are not properly digesting food.
- Red or black poop: This indicates blood in stool.
- Runny stools for more than 2–3 days coupled with fever and/or vomiting.

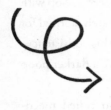

Coughs, Sniffles, Snots—Oh My!

13 Hacks for Baby Colds, Infections, and Immunity

Nothing freaks out a parent more than a sick baby! That feeling you get when you see their temperature spike and hear them coughing and sniffling is one of the most difficult for parents. I can't tell you how many nights I stayed up or had a scare due to high fever, coughing, or a respiratory issue. Not only are babies so little and vulnerable, but also you can't communicate with them and tell them everything will be okay.

Babies, like adults, can get sick for a variety of reasons. They are born with immature immune systems that are still developing, making them more susceptible to all sorts of infections and illnesses. In fact, on average, a healthy baby may experience anywhere from seven to ten colds within their first year. Yes, that's a lot of colds! If your child attends daycare or has an older sibling in school, they might get even more; as they come into contact with new people and places, they become more prone to infections. But all of this is entirely normal. And exposure to germs is an important and natural part of your baby's development and actually helps their immune system strengthen over time. It allows their bodies to learn to recognize and respond to different germs, ultimately building up their immunity for their entire lifetime. Note: It's also important to monitor your baby for complications. While most colds in babies are mild, it's important to watch their symptoms for any of these signs: If your baby develops a high fever, has difficulty breathing, shows signs of dehydration, or if their symptoms worsen or persist for an extended period, please visit a health care professional immediately.

That said, you won't want to rush to the doc for every minor ailment, so it's important to know when it is time to call the doctor and when natural remedies can help. There are many natural ways to help ease baby's symptoms and build up their immunity. (It's well known that antibodies in breast milk can help breastfed babies during the early months, but these maternal antibodies decline over time, and of course, not all parents breastfeed.) Studies show that performing massage consistently on your baby can help boost their immunity and circulation so they are less susceptible to illness.

Research by Tiffany Field found that massage can stimulate the immune system and help your baby fight infections. Also, she found that infant massage decreased autoimmune issues and boosted lung function, helping with respiratory issues.

So while we as parents may feel helpless when baby comes down with yet another cold or cough, remember that there's actually a lot we can do to help them feel better and be on their way to healing. This chapter shares 13 hacks to clear up nasal and chest congestion, tame fever, and help baby to kick that virus.

Hack #1

Down the Hatch

Congestion and snot are a regular part of #newparentlife, but it doesn't have to cause a disruption to your baby's and family's well-being. Facial massage is a great way to relieve congestion or nasal discomfort naturally.

Why It Works

Younger babies need more help with clearing their nasal passageways. This massage will stimulate the sinuses and promote fluid drainage.

Tips

- Make sure to trim your nails so as not to scratch baby's face.
- Babies can be sensitive to their face being touched at first. Get baby used to this sensation by gently touching their face and singing a song while naming their facial features.
- For additional help, I love the NozeBot hospital-grade aspirator to clear out their nose.

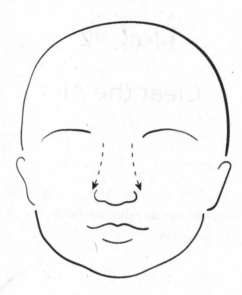

How to Do It

- Use the tips of your fingers to slide down the nasal passageways along the side of the nose.
- Repeat this stroke, making small circular motions and using gentle pressure.
- Repeat ten times.

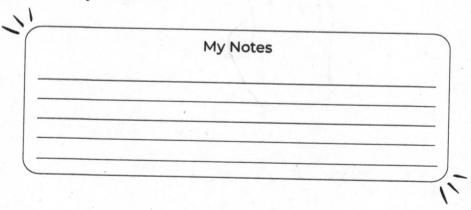

My Notes

Hack #2

Clear the Air

Babies are more prone to nasal congestion and their nostrils are more easily congested due to being smaller in size. Massage can help drain clogged nasal passageways.

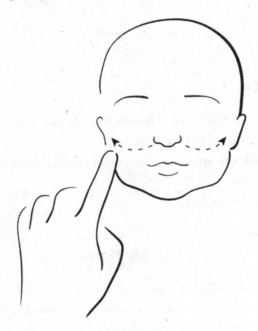

Why It Works

Babies are more prone to nasal congestion due to their smaller anatomy. Doing a lymphatic drainage massage on your baby's face will help promote lymphatic circulation and reduce fluid retention.

Tips

- Watch your baby closely and stop if they are getting uncomfortable.
- If using oil for this massage, only use a tiny drop of organic oil since you don't want baby ingesting it.

How to Do It

- Place your thumbs right at the nostrils and draw out half circles toward the cheeks.
- Use your fingers to stroke right under their cheekbones to help relieve the sinuses.

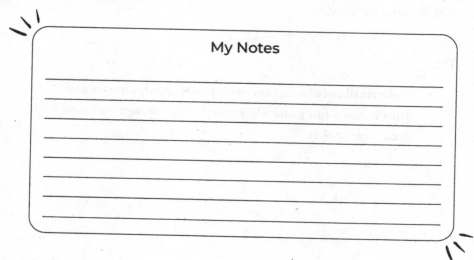

My Notes

Hack #3

Pitter Patter

Few people know that babies are not born with the ability to cough. Chest massage is a wonderful way to help your baby break up mucus in the chest until they master the coughing reflex on their own.

Why It Works

Coughing is a protective reflex that helps clear your baby's nasal passages of irritants and mucus. Babies need time to develop and learn to coordinate the muscles required for coughing. Doing this chest massage will help alleviate fluids in the chest.

Tips

- Make small circular motions with your fingertips in this area.
- Turn it into a fun game while you do this massage action so baby doesn't get restless.'

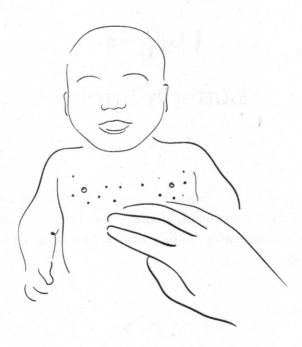

How to Do It

- Use the tips of your fingers to gently tap all over your baby's chest.
- Repeat for 2–3 minutes, singing along to make it a fun experience.

My Notes

Hack #4

Butterfly Stroke

The coughing reflex requires coordination between the diaphragm, throat, and abdominal muscles. Your baby hasn't quite learned how to cough on their own yet, so massaging their chest is a natural way to treat coughs.

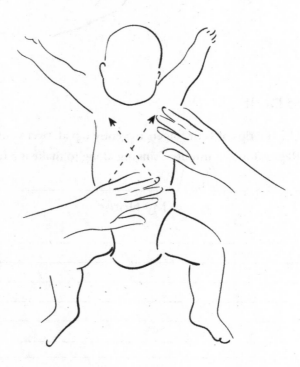

Why It Works

This massage helps promote blood circulation and prepares the muscles for the massage. The Butterfly Stroke is a great way to help your baby relieve mucus and promotes drainage from the upper respiratory system.

Tips

- Use slow and rhythmic movements.
- Be cautious and avoid applying direct pressure on the sternum (breastbone) since it is a sensitive area.

How to Do It

- Use your flat palms and draw your hand from baby's shoulder to right above their rib cage.
- Use the other hand in the same way, and alternate movement of the hands so that one hand is always on baby.
- Repeat for 2 minutes.

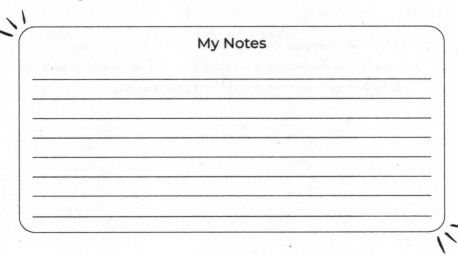

My Notes

Hack #5

Drum Roll

A percussive back massage can work wonders to dislodge trapped fluids in your baby's body. This is a great technique that can be used to help loosen and remove mucus from the lungs.

Why It Works

This can help stimulate coughing, aid in clearing mucus from the airways, and clear respiratory congestion. Many respiratory therapists use vibration/percussive therapy on the back to help clear up fluid from baby's lungs.

Tips

- Make sure you start slow and watch your baby's reactions.
- Gently rub the massager on baby and add additional pressure as baby becomes more comfortable with this sensation.

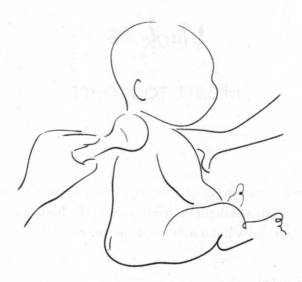

How to Do It

- Sit your baby up and support their chest with one hand.
- Use your Kahlmi baby massager or another gentle vibrating tool to massage baby's upper back.
- You can also lightly tap on your baby's back using the tips of your fingers.

My Notes

Hack #6

Heart to Heart

Continuing a chest massage with the heart stroke is a wonderful way to loosen fluids and drain the lymph nodes. This hack removes congestion in the chest and will instantly bond you and baby.

Why It Works

This gentle heart massage helps clear the lungs of congestion and fluids.

Tip

- Never press too hard on the diaphragm.

How to Do It

- Position your hands with your palms slightly cupped in the middle of your baby's chest.
- Draw a heart with your hands, moving up to the shoulders and ending right at the top of the belly near the diaphragm.
- Use long, slow strokes, repeating three to four times.

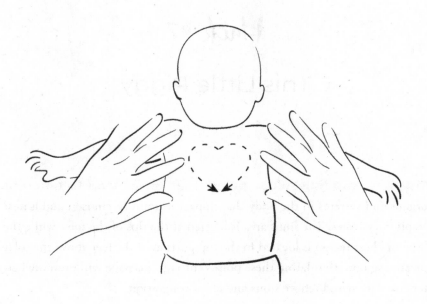

My Notes

_____

_____

_____

_____

_____

_____

_____

_____

Hack #7

This Little Piggy

The feet have reflexology points that correspond to different organs and systems in the body that impact immunity, sinuses, and lungs/ respiratory issues. The sinus area is located at the tips of the toes, while the lung or chest region is located in the top portion of the feet above the solar plexus region. Stimulating these points through massage will promote better circulation and relieve sinus and chest congestion.

Why It Works

Foot reflexology stimulates specific points and sends a message to the brain, which then sends signals to the corresponding organs and systems. This can help to improve circulation, reduce inflammation, and promote healing, as well as relieving congestion.

Tips

- For sinuses, focus on the toes.
- For lung or chest clearing, focus attention on the ball of the foot.
- Recite "This Little Piggy" to engage and stimulate your baby as you massage their toes.

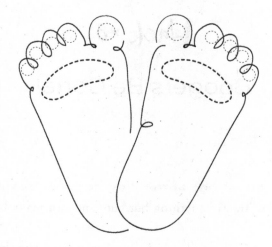

How to Do It

- Use your thumb and index finger to roll the toes gently.
- Hold each toe and press lightly for 5 seconds on each toe. This is great for sinus clearing.
- Massage the upper part of the foot, using your thumbs to glide side to side.

My Notes

Hack #8

Boogers Be Gone!

Nasal congestion is one of the most common symptoms of a cold and viruses. They're anything but cute and can make baby irritable and cranky.

While snot suckers of all kinds do wonders, getting some breast milk in your baby's nose can also help to clear the mucus naturally.

Why It Works

Breast milk has antiviral properties including monolaurin, vitamin A, and lactoferrin. Like saline, breast milk is a buffered liquid, so it won't hurt their delicate nasal passageways.

Tips

- Be careful not to squirt milk up the nose. Try to aim the milk to the side of the nose.
- Do not place dropper deep within the nose. Keep it at the tip of the nose only.
- Try a hospital-grade nasal aspirator like the NozeBot that sucks snot out of baby's nose to help baby.

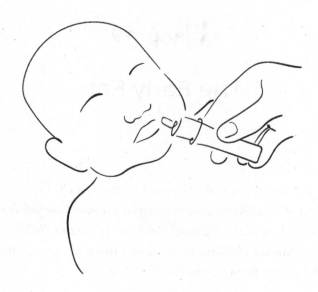

How to Do It

- Lay your baby down on a soft surface.
- Use a dropper to insert a couple drops of breast milk directly into baby's nose.

My Notes

_____
_____
_____
_____
_____
_____
_____
_____

Hack #9

The Early Ears

It's very common for babies and toddlers to get ear infections, with five out of six children experiencing an ear infection before their third birthday according to the National Institutes of Health. While many doctors will recommend antibiotics, you can try this massage technique to help with fluid drainage from the middle ear.

Why It Works

The Eustachian tube connects the upper throat to the middle ear and is smaller in children, making it more difficult for fluid to drain out of the ear. This massage works by massaging the Eustachian tube and helping the fluid drain.

Tips

- Use a warm compress after the massage, making sure no water gets in the ears.
- If the ear infection doesn't clear up in a few days, make sure to see a doctor.
- Ear infections and fevers can often go hand in hand, with 50 percent of babies experiencing fevers alongside ear infections. If your child has a persistent low-grade fever lasting more than 2 days, make sure to see a doctor to find out if an ear infection is causing it.

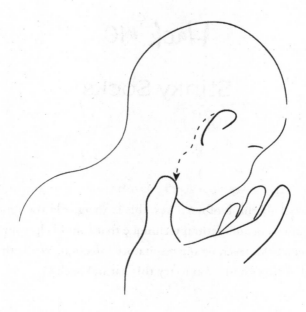

How to Do It

- Add a little edible-grade, organic coconut or jojoba oil to your thumb.
- Find the spot between the back of your child's infected ear and the bone behind the ear and apply gentle pressure with your thumb.
- Using medium to firm pressure, slide your thumb down the neck to the collarbone.

My Notes

Hack #10

Stinky Socks

Onions in baby's socks? You're probably thinking: Now what will this crazy lady think of next! Yes, this is an age-old tradition, but it is actually an amazing and natural technique that could help your baby next time they get a cold, fever, or any respiratory infection. While the evidence is anecdotal, it won't harm you to try this natural hack.

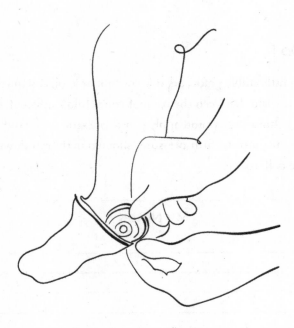

Why It Works

Onions are antiviral, antibacterial, and antifungal. When you place slices of onion on the bottoms of the feet, folklore tells us that the feet will absorb the onion juice to kill off whatever is causing the fever. The sulfur in the onion will also help to draw out mucus and fluids if your baby is showing signs of an illness.

Tips

- Never leave the onions in their socks overnight.
- Remove the onions and socks after a maximum of 20 minutes.
- This also works for older kids and adults!

How to Do It

- Cut a few slices of red or white onion.
- Place in baby's socks for 15–20 minutes.

My Notes

Hack #11

Fever No More

When baby gets a fever, it can be a scary experience for a parent—but occasional illness and fevers do come with the territory. While many doctors used to warn that untreated fevers can be dangerous, the American Academy of Pediatrics now says that most fevers (especially low-grade fevers) do not necessarily need to be treated with Tylenol or Motrin but can instead be allowed to run their course.

Why It Works

Many studies have shown that acupressure can relieve inflammation in the body and help the body fight off infections naturally. Stimulating this point (LU11, in acupuncture and acupressure) helps the body relieve body aches associated with fevers.

Tip

- Make cucumber juice to reduce the fever naturally by blending a cucumber and feeding it to your baby (1 month+) with a feeding syringe or in a bottle.

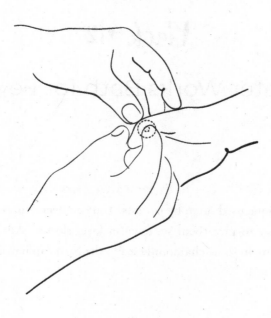

How to Do It

- Find the point just under your baby's thumbnail on the radial side (outside) of the digit.
- Gently press this point for 10–20 seconds without squeezing.
- Repeat every 2–3 hours until the temperature drops.

My Notes

Hack #12

Water Works Bath for Fever

Using lukewarm baths to draw down fever is a wonderful and natural technique used often by parents. You can even climb into the bath with your baby to give them some extra love, skin-to-skin contact, and support. Adding in some chamomile tea to the bath can naturally draw the fever down as well.

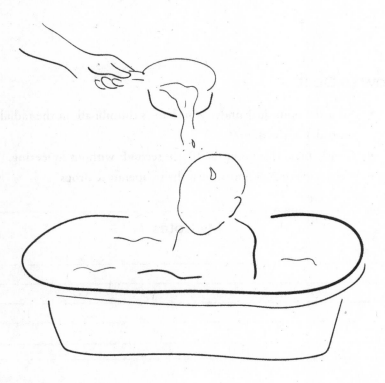

Why It Works

While many parents want to cool down baby quickly using a colder bath temperature, it can actually cause baby to shiver and will increase their core body temperature.

Tips

- Provide extra liquids by nursing often and giving your baby more formula to keep them hydrated.
- Never put a feverish child into cold water. It will bring the fever down too fast and could cause a febrile seizure.

How to Do It

- Draw a lukewarm bath for you and your baby. Make sure it is not too warm or cold with a temperature between 90°F and 95°F (use a bath thermometer to check).
- Place your baby in a baby tub in the bath and then join them in the bath.
- Remove your baby from the tub and place them on your chest as you sink into the lukewarm water. Soak in the water 5–15 minutes.
- You can also do a lukewarm sponge bath with baby in the baby tub.

My Notes

_____

_____

_____

_____

_____

Hack #13

Medicine Go Down!

Baby won't take their meds? While most babies should not take medication unless under strict doctor's orders, there are times when you will want to give them a little gripe water to help with gas, or a pain reliever if they are teething or if their fever gets too high. Not a problem with this easy and natural hack.

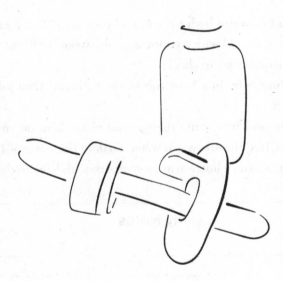

Why It Works

Babies tend to feel more comfortable when they are nursing and have a familiar object to suck on rather than a medicine dispenser. This technique cuts out the tears while helping you deliver their medication.

Tip

- Always speak to your pediatrician before giving baby any medication.

How to Do It

- Remove a nipple from your baby's favorite bottle.
- Place the medicine dispenser in the nipple and hold it to your baby's mouth.
- Let them suck the medicine out through the nipple.

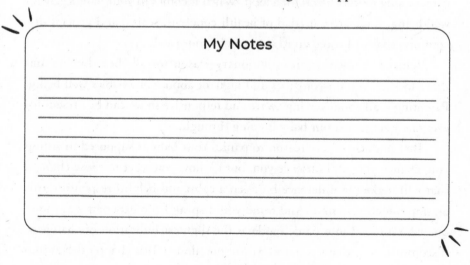

My Notes

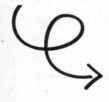

Daily Maintenance

11 Hacks for Teething, Skin Care, and Bathing

Just when you have figured out how to soothe your baby and think you are getting the hang of this parenting thing, some new challenge comes along to knock you for a loop. When it comes to your baby's general well-being, there are a myriad of health concerns, scares, and general discomforts that will come up to stop you in your tracks.

Remember, there is an evolutionary reason for all these hitches and that's to keep you on your toes and vigilant about your baby's well-being. Parenting is all about staying aware and responsive so we can be present for every new stage that our baby is going through.

That said, there's no reason to panic. Your baby is supposed to stump you, change you, and unsettle you, but it's how you react to those changes that will make the difference between a calm and helpful response versus an unproductive frenzy. (And mind you, I speak from experience as someone who jumped into panic mode at the slightest indication of change or discomfort, so if that's you, too, you're not alone!) This chapter delves into those concerns that can come up from day to day—from teething pain to skin issues and even just making bath time better.

And there's a reason I'm spending so much of this chapter talking about baths. As a new mom, I always looked forward to bath time. Bath time is the great daily equalizer in a parent's life. It is a sign that nighttime is approaching, when the two of you will (hopefully) finally get a little sleep and can wind down the day. Many consider the bathing process the light at the end of the proverbial baby care daily tunnel.

While some babies love and look forward to bath time as much as we parents do, others aren't so keen on water play. There are many ways to bathe your baby, with many parents preferring sink tubs in the first month so they can bathe their baby in comfort. Plush sink tubs from Blooming Bath and Skip Hop can be a great way to keep your baby cozy while helping get baby comfortable in the water. (Remember, you won't want to bathe your baby before their umbilical stump falls off, which usually takes 1–2 weeks. During that time, only give light sponge baths.) Bath time is also a great time to incorporate baby massage, as baby is already more relaxed and can enjoy the benefits of a short massage while luxuriating in their bath. The other benefits of regular bath times include keeping your baby's skin barrier healthy and free of rashes and dryness. Bathing also stimulates the vagus nerve, which changes brain waves and slows the heart rate to promote relaxation before nighttime sleep. And the routine of a bath time every night (no need for soap or shampoos more than once a week) helps to signal that it's time for bed.

This section will help you find ways to inject the most nurturing and care into your daily routine to help your baby with a variety of issues, from teething to cradle cap and eczema.

Hack #1

Gum Massage

Teething is a gradual process. It can take 5–33 months to get through the full teething journey, but don't worry, your baby will only have teething pain for a week during each eruption. Of course, when you're going through the teething stage and baby is irritable, fussy, and crying, it can feel like a never-ending process. Massage for teething pain can be a helpful way to soothe your baby and make the process a little easier.

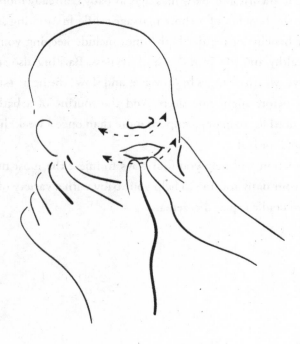

Why It Works

Sore, swollen, and inflamed gums are a natural byproduct of the teething process. Applying pressure with your fingers to the gum line can counter the pressure of the teeth breaking through.

Tips

- Sing or talk gently to your baby during the massage to relax them.
- Be patient and calm as some babies take time to adjust to their face being massaged.
- Follow the massage with a chilled teether they can chew on.

How to Do It

- Place your baby in a comfortable position lying down on a soft surface.
- Use clean fingers to massage the mouth area at the upper lip and beneath the lower lip. You don't need to put your fingers in your baby's mouth. This can be done simply by massaging the outer lip areas that cover the gums.
- Use gentle strokes and make small circles to make sure you are massaging their gum line.

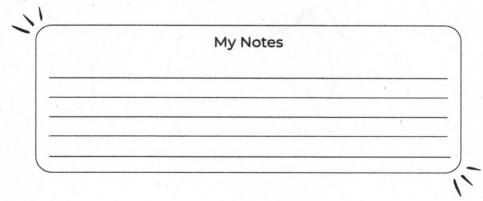

My Notes

Hack #2

Jaw Soother

Teething is never one and done. It can be a drawn-out process and eruptions can take you by surprise. Some signs your child is teething include excessive drooling, low-grade fevers, and general crankiness. Teething is a long process, but you can make it easier by learning to massage your baby's cheeks and gum area.

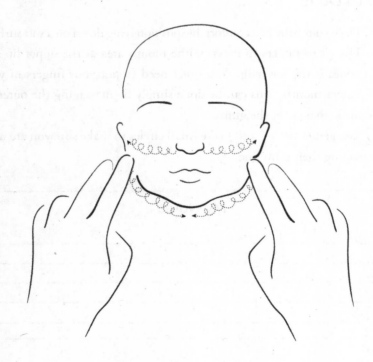

Why It Works

Massaging your baby's cheeks and jaw can be a helpful way to soothe your baby and make the teething process a little easier. It can reduce tension and pressure brought about by teething and will relax them.

Tip

- Offer your baby cold frozen foods like mashed bananas or apple slices from the freezer to soothe their gums.

How to Do It

- Place two fingers at the base of your child's ears on both sides of their head.
- Use your fingers to draw small circles along the jawline down the chin. Repeat three to four times.
- Massage your baby's cheeks by placing your fingers on their cheeks by the base of their nose and drawing small circles outward to the top of their ears.
- Repeat the sequence three to five times.

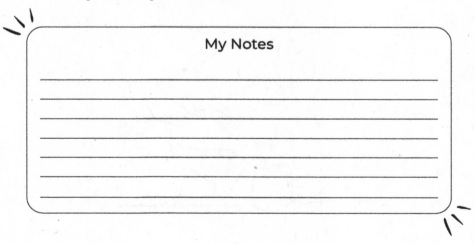

My Notes

Hack #3

Natural Teething Rx

Did you know you can significantly decrease teething pain with ingredients you already have in your home? Here's one way to help reduce the pain with an ordinary chamomile tea from your pantry.

Why It Works

Chamomile tea is a natural remedy that has been used for centuries to soothe a variety of ailments, including teething pain. The anti-inflammatory and calming properties of chamomile can help to reduce gum inflammation and ease discomfort.

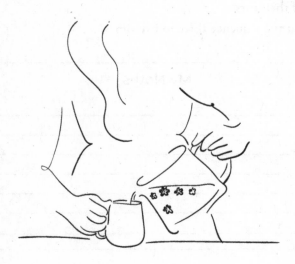

Tips

- For babies 6 months+, you can make chamomile popsicles to numb their sore gums and provide teething relief.
- Make sure to thoroughly cool the tea before giving it to your baby.

How to Do It

- Make some hot chamomile tea and then cool it in the fridge.
- Clean your finger, then dip it into the chamomile tea and rub on your baby's gum line.
- You can also just cool the tea in the freezer and give your baby a small amount on a spoon.

My Notes

_____
_____
_____
_____
_____
_____
_____
_____

Hack #4

Jaundice Hack

Like my firstborn, many babies will experience jaundice in the first month of their life, about 60–80 percent of all babies. While photo-therapy lights can help, a simple daily baby massage routine can help them as well.

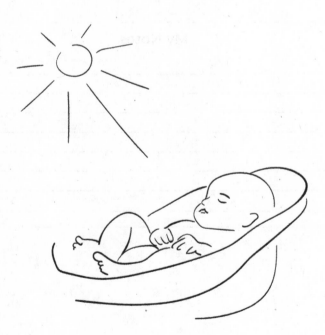

Why It Works

A few recent studies show that infant massage can reduce levels of bilirubin, the compound that causes jaundice. Baby massage also increases the frequency of bowel movements, which does wonders for removing excess bilirubin from the body.

Tips

- Some sun is okay, but don't leave your baby in direct sunlight for any length of time.
- Always massage their belly to help them poop, which helps with jaundice.

How to Do It

- Start with a full baby massage every morning and night.
- Repeat the massage ritual every day.
- Try to give your baby much indirect natural light, leaving them by a window for 15–20 minutes a day to soak up the sun's rays.

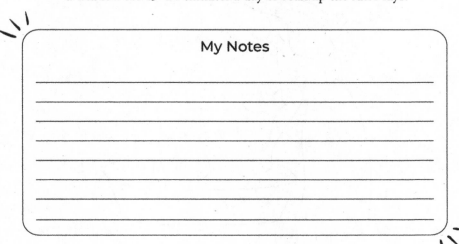

My Notes

Hack #5

Oatmeal Bath

You might be surprised to learn that a simple breakfast ingredient from your pantry can help your baby with everything from eczema to skin/diaper rash, and even baby acne. Oatmeal!

Why It Works

Colloidal oats are oats ground into a very fine powder. This allows the oatmeal to penetrate and act as a calming emollient to soothe and moisturize dry and irritated skin.

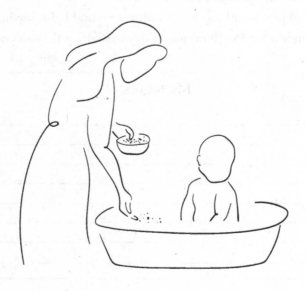

Tips

- Do *not* use soaps or shampoos since this bath is intended to moisturize baby's skin.
- Be careful when handling baby after an oatmeal bath as it makes baby super slippery.
- Do not rinse baby after the bath. Just towel off as usual.

How to Do It

- Place a cup of dry oats into a blender or coffee grinder and process until it turns into a fine powder.
- Mix the ground oats into a running lukewarm baby bath.
- Keep mixing the oats with the water until the bath has a milky appearance.
- Place baby in supervised bath for 10–20 minutes.

My Notes

_____
_____
_____
_____
_____
_____
_____
_____

Hack #6

Curb Cradle Cap

More annoying than worrisome, cradle cap is a very common skin condition in babies that creates rough patches and scaly scalp conditions. Cradle cap is harmless and usually goes away on its own within a few weeks or months, but that doesn't mean you can't treat it at home using simple ingredients. A simple head massage before bathing can be an amazing way to massage your baby and form new neural pathways while treating their cradle cap.

Why It Works

Scientists have yet to figure out the causes of cradle cap (also known as infantile seborrheic dermatitis). Some believe it is tied to hormonal shifts in the mother and others point to yeast known as *Malassezia* that grows in sebum. Coconut oil is considered antifungal, which helps to control the yeast.

Tips

- To make your own shampoo, mix ¼ cup castile soap and 1 teaspoon organic, edible-grade coconut oil with ¾ cup distilled water.
- Limit how much you shampoo baby's scalp as it removes the natural oils from the skin and can cause an overproduction of the scalp's sebum, making cradle cap even worse.
- Never pick the flakes off. Your baby's head is extremely sensitive.

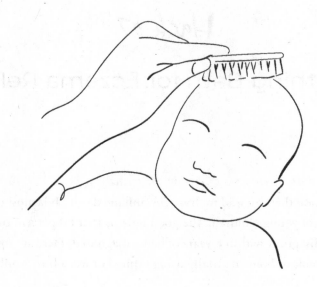

How to Do It

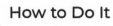

- Massage a thin coat of edible-grade, organic coconut or jojoba oil into baby's scalp.
- Let it sit for 20–30 minutes.
- Use a soft-bristle baby brush to gently brush off the flakes.
- Rinse scalp as usual and follow with homemade gentle hair shampoo (see the tips for my favorite recipe).

My Notes

_____
_____
_____
_____
_____

Hack #7

Soothing Bath for Eczema Relief

Eczema, also known as atopic dermatitis, is a very common skin condition that can lead to dry, itchy, inflamed skin. It is most common in babies and young children. The good news is that 80 percent of eczema cases will disappear within 8 years of being diagnosed. Here are some ways to treat eczema at home naturally using expired or extra breast milk.

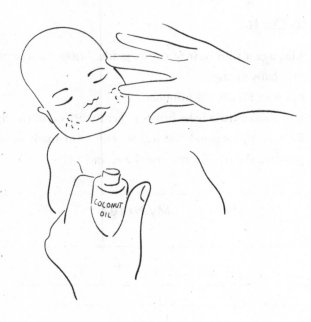

Why It Works

Breast milk has been shown to help soothe and treat inflammation caused by eczema and works wonders on sensitive, irritation-prone baby skin.

Tip

- You can also use breast milk during the day, rather than just at bath time, to treat eczema: just dab some milk on a cotton ball and apply directly to affected area.

How to Do It

- Fill your baby's bath with lukewarm water.
- Mix in ½ cup breast milk until the water turns cloudy.
- Allow your baby to soak in the bath for 5–20 minutes.
- Use a washcloth to spread the milky mixture all over their body.
- Pat dry and use unrefined organic coconut oil to seal in the benefits.

My Notes

Hack #8

Pimple Cure

One of the most surprising conditions parents see in babies is baby acne. Some babies are born with small pimples all over their face while others can develop acne from 2 weeks to 1 year of age. For newborn babies with acne (about 20 percent of all babies), it usually goes away within a matter of 2 weeks, but if it persists, you can try some of the natural tips below.

Why It Works

Hormones from mom are still circulating in baby's body and are often the cause of baby acne. (Sorry, moms—as if we moms didn't get enough blame already!) That's why breast milk is so wonderful to use as it is antibacterial and can be used on mom's or dad's skin as well to help soothe outbreaks.

Tips

- Don't use soap, oil, or other adult products on baby's face.
- Never try to touch or rub the pimples with your fingers as this can lead to infection.

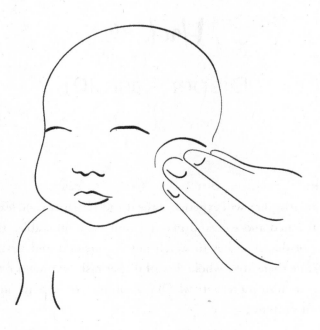

How to Do It

- Start by cleaning your baby's face two times a day with warm water and a washcloth. Gently dry by patting their face.
- Use cotton balls soaked in breast milk to gently pat their face. Let air dry.

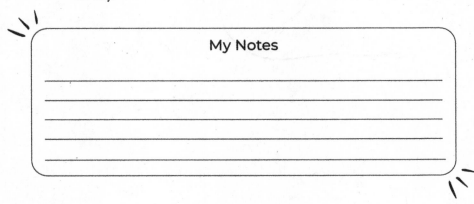

My Notes

Hack #9

Diaper Rash 101

Sometimes despite your best efforts to change your baby's diaper regularly, they will experience the dreaded diaper rash, leaving their bottoms irritated and sore and making your baby miserable. There are a few types of diaper rashes to watch out for: irritant and yeast (fungal) rashes. While there are a whole slew of diaper rash ointments on the market, there are also more natural DIY solutions you can try at home to soothe their bottoms.

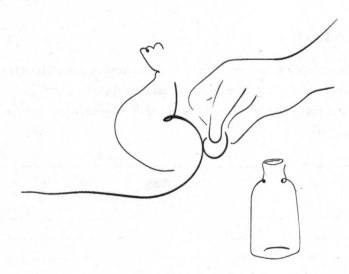

Why It Works

Breast milk and coconut oil have natural anti-inflammatory properties and have been shown to help with common irritant infections, while coconut oil can provide an extra skin barrier. Apple cider vinegar is a fermented liquid that eliminates bacteria and hinders the growth of yeast.

Tips

- Change your baby's diaper frequently.
- Always let their bottom air dry for as long as possible.
- Avoid using wipes as they can irritate baby's skin.

Irritant Diaper Rash

This is the most common type of diaper rash and looks like a light pink irritation on baby's bottom. This is caused by wearing a diaper too long and/or having infrequent changes. A natural solution for this is either coconut oil, breast milk, or an oatmeal bath (see page 178) in the morning and evening.

Yeast Diaper Rash

Irritation caused by yeast is usually a brighter red rash that can include small bumps and pimples. This can be treated by diluting 2 tablespoons of apple cider vinegar in a small bowl of water and using a cotton ball to gently swab the solution onto your baby's body.

My Notes

_____

_____

Hack #10

The No-Stress Bath

Swaddle bathing is a relatively new practice around the world and is becoming more widely accepted in neonatal hospital settings. Traditional baths can be difficult for some babies, leading to stressful associations with water and loss of heat during the bath. This practice is best started after your baby's umbilical cord falls off as you can't get this part wet.

Why It Works

A 2014 study found that babies who are swaddled during the bath tend to stay warmer, cry less, and remain calmer than with traditional bathing techniques.

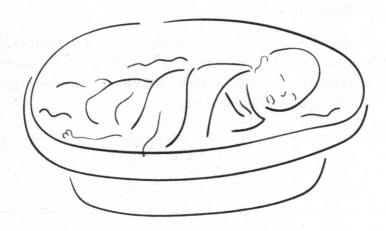

Tips

- Never leave baby unattended in the bath.
- Always make sure the water is a comfortable warm temperature not to exceed 95°F. Test the water with a bath thermometer or your wrist.

How to Do It

- Fill a small sink tub with warm water.
- Swaddle your baby in a large fleece blanket, as the fleece doesn't retain as much moisture as other blankets and maintains heat better. Make sure you swaddle loosely so you can wrap and unwrap baby to maintain warmth.
- Take out their arms and legs one at a time, wash, and then place back into the swaddle.
- Unwrap their torso and chest and wash with the sides of the blanket.

My Notes

_____
_____
_____
_____
_____
_____
_____
_____

Hack #11

Here's Water in Your Eye

For so long, we have been taught to keep water out of our baby's faces and eyes because it can startle and upset them. There are even baby bath visors and special waterspouts that are used to keep soap and shampoo out of their eyes. But introducing water on baby's face is an infant bathing technique that can actually reduce their fear of the water and prepare your baby for swimming lessons.

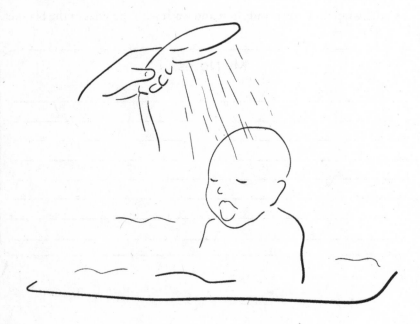

Why It Works

Ask any swim instructor and they will tell you that babies have a hard time getting their faces wet. This hack has parents introduce water on the face in a safe and gentle way.

Tips

- If your baby starts crying or is visibly upset, stop and try another time.
- Make sure to not get water in baby's ears; if water enters the ear it can increase the risk of ear infection.

How to Do It

- Tell your baby what you are about to do: "I am pouring water on your head and face."
- Start slowly. Trickle small amounts of water on the top of their head and down the back.
- Wipe the water off their eyes and face using a washcloth.

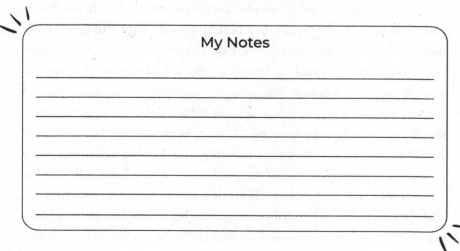

My Notes

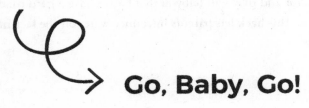

Go, Baby, Go!
19 Hacks for Motor and Brain Development

In this book's previous chapters, we uncovered the myriad of ways infant massage can help your baby, including relieving common colds, teething pain, constipation, and fevers; improving sleep; and of course, increasing bonding. But did you know baby massage hacks and other natural bodywork techniques can also help your baby grow and develop physically and cognitively?

Baby massage has numerous physical developmental benefits for babies and toddlers, including promoting healthy growth, aiding in gross motor skills, and even helping with delays. Parents and caregivers can also incorporate other exercises such as stretching, yoga, and tummy time to promote physical development. Water massage and baby spas are other fun and effective ways to promote motor skills in babies. Baby massage and gentle stretching can help to increase muscle tone, improve range of motion and flexibility, and assist with sitting, crawling, and walking milestones. Baby massage also helps to stimulate the production of new brain cells and the formation of new neural connections that are the pathways that help the brain process information. Baby massage has been shown to increase blood flow to the brain, which provides the brain with the oxygen and nutrients it needs to grow and develop.

There have been many studies showing the importance of baby massage for motor, cognitive, and speech development. For instance, researchers in Istanbul discovered that when mothers massaged their babies 15 minutes a day, fine motor, gross motor, and speech skill development was significantly higher than in the non-massaged group. Another study, published in the journal *Infant Behavior and Development*, showed that babies who received daily massage during a 2-year period had much higher Mental Development Index (MDI) scores than the non-massage control group.

All this being said, remember: *Every baby is different and will reach their developmental milestones at their own pace.* As your baby grows in your belly, they are already developing muscle strength and coordination as they stretch and kick. Motor development will continue after birth and talk of milestones often makes parents anxious as they make comparisons and size up their baby's fitness to others.

"Her baby is already walking. My baby is not!"

"Look at that baby climbing. My baby can barely crawl."

As someone who had to seek out occupational and physical therapy for my kids at an early age, I know that there are certain times we need to give our kids a little boost, but that is no reason to get hung up on some arbitrary milestone calendar. That said, if you do feel your baby has delays or other issues like torticollis or flat head, you should speak to your pediatrician and combine at-home exercises with professional help.

When it comes to brain development, studies have shown that motor and brain development work in tandem. We've all heard about the mind/body connection and your baby's development is no exception. All the interaction and massage you have learned will do wonders for your baby's growing brain.

Hack #1

Back Massage

I love back massages because you're really accomplishing two things: (1) Helping your baby get tummy time; (2) Developing strength in their neck, back, and shoulders that will help them climb and crawl.

Why It Works

Back massage is extremely relaxing for babies and will help them log more tummy-time minutes, especially if you place a mirror or toys in front of them.

Tips

- Prop your baby up on a bolster or a rolled towel/blanket to make your baby more comfortable and give them additional support.
- Never place pressure on the spine directly.

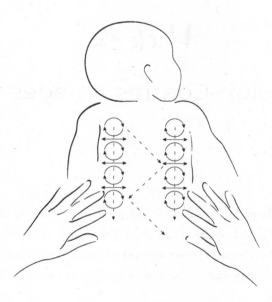

How to Do It

- Start with long, smooth strokes using your fingers and palms to relax your baby for the massage.
- Make small circles down each side of their back, avoiding the spinal column.
- Use the flat side of your palms to make a zigzag pattern across your baby's back.
- Massage their bum using firm circular strokes.

My Notes

Hack #2

High-Contrast Images

At birth and for a few months after, babies don't see us very clearly (think large faceless blobs) and need more time to develop their visual skills. Clinical research has shown that high-contrast images help them develop their focus. High-contrast images are a great way to help your baby's visual development, so be sure to give them plenty of opportunities to look at them.

Why It Works

Clinical research has shown that bold black-and-white high-contrast images help babies develop their focus and stimulate the optic nerves. Engagement with contrasting images and with diverse textures and patterns boosts infants' learning and focus.

Tips

- While all you really need for tummy time is a comfortable mat, you can also place baby in a developmentally approved gym like Lovevery's.
- Another great hack is to attach a rear-facing car seat toy like Taf Toys' to engage your baby while on the road.

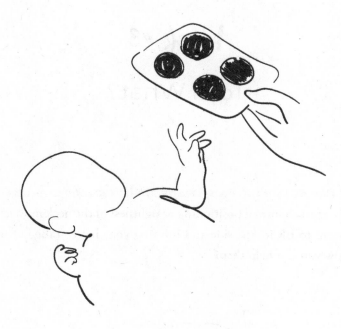

How to Do It

- Keep the cards about 8–11 inches away from baby's face as that is the range they can see best in the early months.
- Switch flash cards every 10–20 seconds. Or, you can simply prop a few cards where baby can see them and catch a few minutes to relax!
- Use cards and other black, white, and red visual cues to keep baby occupied during tummy time.

My Notes

_____

_____

_____

Hack #3

Torti What?

Ever notice that your baby leans their head in one direction?
Torticollis is an abnormal positioning or tightness of the neck muscles, causing the head to tilt to one side and limiting your baby's range of motion. Here's how you can help them.

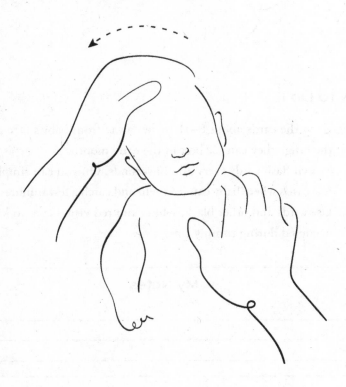

Why It Works

Torticollis usually occurs in the first 3–6 months but can also show up later. Most babies with torticollis get better through position changes and stretching exercises. But be patient since it takes up to 6 months to treat.

 ## Tips

- Repeat this stretch and massage multiple times a day, gradually increasing your baby's range of motion over time.
- Always watch baby's reactions when stretching to ensure they are comfortable.
- Encourage additional time so baby can strengthen their neck muscles.

 ## How to Do It

- Sit your baby upright on your lap.
- Hold a desired object to the side and have them turn their head to increase range of motion.
- Stretch the neck muscles by gently turning baby's head to the affected side and holding it in that position for a few seconds.
- Use your hand to gently massage the affected side, working on the neck and shoulders, and repeat this stretch five times.

My Notes

_____

_____

_____

Hack #4

Who You Calling Flat Head?

It's amazing all the things parents have to worry about. As a new mom, I had no idea that flat head syndrome was even a thing. Flat head syndrome, also known as positional plagiocephaly, is a condition where a baby's head develops a flat spot. It happens because our babies tend to lie down in the same position, whether on their side or on their back, for prolonged periods of time. Here's a hack to counteract this.

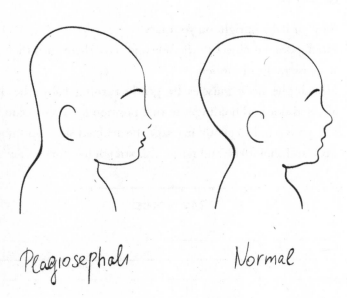

Plagiosephali   Normal

Why It Works

At birth, the bones in a baby's skull are soft and malleable, which makes them mold to the shape of the surface they are lying on. If a baby spends too much time lying in the same position, the bones on the side of the head that are in contact with the surface will begin to flatten over time. While most cases clear up by 2 years of age, some will require more physical therapy including wearing a helmet.

Tips

- Long periods of time in swings and other baby "container devices" can lead to flat head. If you need to lay baby down, try to alternate the setting so they can enjoy a variety of positions.
- Carry your baby in a carrier when you are able, as this can relieve pressure on their skull from lying down.
- I love the Tushbaby hip carrier to keep baby upright and give parents some back relief.

How to Do It

- Allow for plenty of tummy time to keep baby off their back.
- Help your baby adjust their head position by placing high-stimulation items (black, white, and red designed cards and toys) on alternate sides to encourage them to switch positions.

My Notes

_____

_____

_____

Hack #5

Tummy Time

Tummy time is one of the most important activities for babies to engage in. But that doesn't mean they have to like it. In fact, many babies will cry and scream the entire time at first, so don't let that discourage you. Here are some goals for tummy time, based on guidance from the AAP and prominent children's hospitals.

- Newborns: Start with 1–2 minutes of tummy time, 4–5 times a day, every day. Gradually increase the length of each tummy-time session.
- By 7 weeks: Try for 20–30 minutes of tummy time per day.
- By 4 months: Ramp up their tummy time to up to 90 minutes per day.

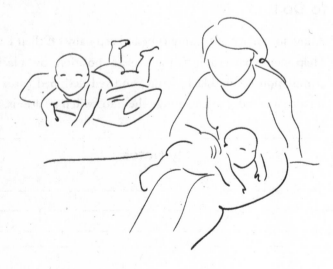

Why It Works

Tummy time is important for babies because it helps to develop their head, neck, and upper body strength, which ultimately prepares them to roll over, crawl, and walk.

Tips

- For newborns, carrying your baby in a sling and letting them rest on your chest on their tummy counts as tummy time.
- As kids get older, you will want to place them on their tummy on a soft surface. Make sure to place fun objects for them to grasp and reach for.
- For babies who don't love tummy time, place them on top of a bolster or a Boppy-like pillow to give them a little support on their chest.
- If baby's arms move to the side, position their arms beneath them so they can get more support.
- If your baby gets fussy, take a break and try again later, as you want them to have a positive association with tummy time.

How to Do It

- Place your baby on a soft blanket or mat.
- Put some interesting toys within reach of your baby.
- Get down to eye level with your baby, then talk and sing to them while they're on their tummy.

My Notes

_____

_____

Hack #6

Super Baby

For babies who don't love tummy time, finding new ways to get them on their tummy is crucial. I love this exercise because it is not only fun for baby and provides direct eye and physical contact, it is also wonderful for the parent as a way to release stress.

Why It Works

Offering more tummy time through engaging play can decrease restlessness associated with solo tummy floor time and will increase your baby's balance, as well as muscle strength and tone.

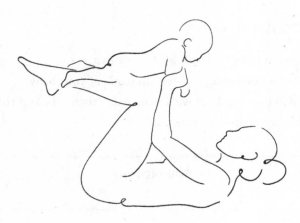

Tips

- Always hold on tightly to your baby during this exercise.
- Make sure to hold your baby's eye contact.
- Use your voice to make fun flying noises to keep baby engaged.

How to Do It

- Lie on your back with your knees bent at a 90-degree angle.
- Place your baby with their stomach on your shins, holding their shoulders or hips tightly.
- Slowly, with your legs bent and balancing baby on top, move your legs up and down.
- Rock back and forth, gently making a fun swooshing noise.

My Notes

Hack #7

Baecycles

Cycling your baby's legs is a common move used for constipation and gas, but did you know it's also a wonderful way to strengthen your baby's knees, hips, and legs, and increase flexibility? It even develops their core abdominal muscles, which helps them with a variety of developmental milestones. You should also cycle their arms to build strength and improve range of motion in the shoulders and elbow joints.

Why It Works

This exercise improves your baby's range of motion, helps with digestion, and strengthens arm and leg muscles.

Tips

- Start slow and gentle with baby and see how they react.
- Sing "The Wheels on the Bus" or any upbeat song to make this a fun activity while you move their arms and legs in time to the music.

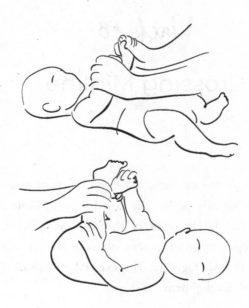

How to Do It

- Place your baby on their back.
- Take one foot gently into each of your hands.
- Start cycling your baby's legs. Continue for 2–3 minutes.
- Move baby's legs together and straighten them.
- Repeat the same motion with their arms.

My Notes

Hack #8

Crossing Midline

If you're not a physical or occupational therapist, the concept of crossing the midline may be entirely new for you. While most parents won't even notice the development of this vital skill, it's important to encourage its development using specific exercises that encourage baby to use both sides of their body together. This exercise will also help with brain and social/emotional development.

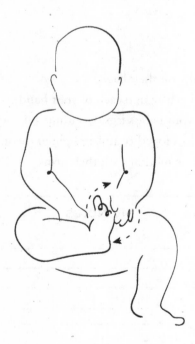

Why It Works

Crossing the midline is an essential part of helping to develop basic gross and fine motor skills, allowing your baby to learn how to use both sides of the body in tandem, which is called bilateral coordination. Crossing the midline takes extra processing time. By engaging your child in activities that encourage crossing the midline, you may also be helping to train their brain.

Tips

- Try placing items in an arc in front of your baby and have them reach for them across their body.
- Hand clapping is also a crossing midline activity, so practice this skill with them early on by singing songs and clapping your hands to encourage them to mimic you.

How to Do It

- Lay baby down comfortably on the floor.
- Hold one of baby's arms in one hand and their opposite foot in your other hand.
- Gently draw the opposite arm and leg together, allowing the foot and arm to make contact.
- Repeat five times before switching to the other side.

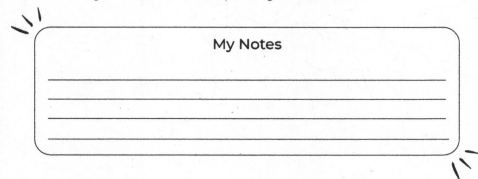

My Notes

Hack #9

Up, Up, and Away

Lifting your baby's arms up, down, and to the side is not only a fun game but has many developmental benefits that will help them coordinate and strengthen their shoulder and neck muscles.

Why It Works

These exercises are all about building strength and increasing the range of motion in your baby's shoulders and arms.

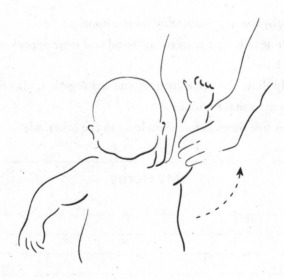

Tips

- Never raise or stretch your baby's arms past their natural range of motion.
- Hold their shoulder as you glide their arm up and to the side.
- Repeat these exercises several times a day, making it a fun game for them.

How to Do It

- Lay your baby on a soft mat or rug or on a changing table.
- Holding their wrist, gently lift one arm up at a time to meet their head.
- Alternate lifting arms, making sure not to exceed their natural range of movement. Do this five times with each arm.
- Raise and lower both arms at the same time.

My Notes

_____
_____
_____
_____
_____
_____
_____
_____

Hack #10

Peekaboo (It's Not Just Child's Play)

Playing peekaboo may seem like a silly little game, but it's actually a great way to help your baby learn object permanence.

Why It Works

Peekaboo is great for helping babies develop object permanence, which is an understanding that an object still exists even when you can't see it. This skill helps baby feel secure and reduces attachment anxiety. Peekaboo also encourages baby to track your movements and develop their eye-hand coordination.

Tips

- Make sure not to startle your baby.
- Always say "Where are you?" when you hide and "Peekaboo!" or "I see you!" when you reveal yourself so they know it's a fun game.
- Be expressive and animated when you play peekaboo. This will help your baby stay engaged.
- Repeat the game several times since babies love repetition.

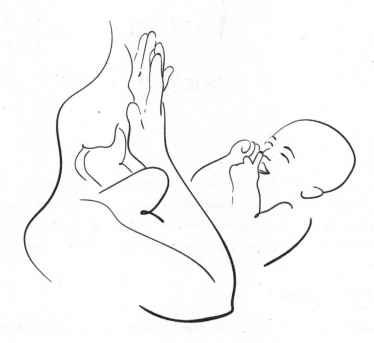

How to Do It

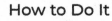

- Get a scarf and place it in front of your face to "hide."
- Move the scarf to show your face, saying "Peekaboo!" in a fun voice.
- You can also play the game by hiding behind a sofa or counter and popping up.

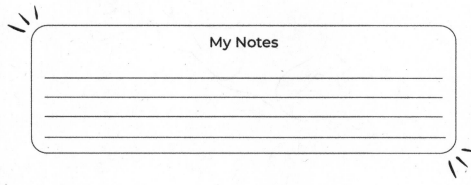

My Notes

Hack #11

Kick It!

Ever notice your baby's desire to kick their legs, whether it was in utero or out in the real world? That's because kicking strengthens their hip and leg muscles, preparing them for rolling and crawling. You can do daily exercises to help your baby develop and strengthen these vital muscles.

Why It Works

Pushing away with the legs increases the strength and range of motion in your baby's legs.

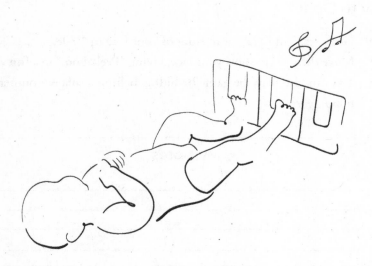

Tip

- Don't force this exercise, as babies will naturally want to push their legs against something. If it's not working today, try again another day.

How to Do It

- Place a piano toy at the foot of baby's bed or crib and let them push against the toy and delight in the sounds they create.
- If you don't have a piano, place your baby on their back and place your palm against your baby's foot to offer resistance as they push forward.

My Notes

_____

_____

_____

_____

_____

_____

_____

Hack #12

Baby Crunches

Who doesn't want their baby to have a six-pack? I'm kidding, of course, but in all seriousness, baby's core strength is so important as a foundation for later activities such as rolling over, sitting up unassisted, and walking. But make sure your baby is ready. While some babies are ready at 4 months, others will need more time.

Why It Works

There are many physical benefits that come from having a strong core, but developing strong baby abs also has a number of cognitive and social benefits. There is a strong connection between cognitive and motor development. With a strong core, your baby is more likely to be able to focus and pay attention, which can help them to learn and develop. They are also more likely to be able to interact with other people and play with toys, which can assist with softer social skills.

Tips

- Your baby should be able to support their own head before attempting this activity.
- Support your baby's back as you lift them.
- Be gentle as you draw them up so as not to put too much pressure on their neck and shoulders.

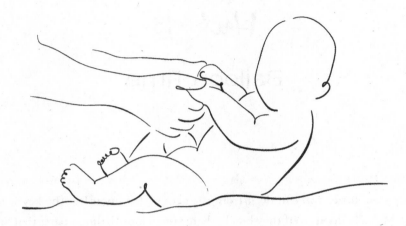

How to Do It

- Lay your baby on a play mat on their back.
- Hold both of your baby's hands and slowly and gently pull up your baby to a sitting position.
- Your baby will start to lift their head and crunch their belly as they get a little higher.
- Lower them to the floor and repeat a few times.

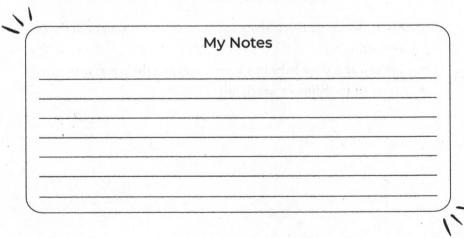

My Notes

Hack #13

Balloon Time

I love this exercise and wish I had done it with my babies when they were little. You can do it from the ages of 1–8 months. The key is to use Mylar balloons so if they break, there are no loose balloon parts that are a danger to babies.

Why It Works

The cause and effect coupled with the high-contrast balloons will captivate their attention, help improve eye tracking, and encourage them to exercise their muscles.

Tips

- Always supervise this activity so baby doesn't get caught in the balloon strings.
- You can also place baby in a bouncer during the activity.
- Never tie the balloons too tightly.

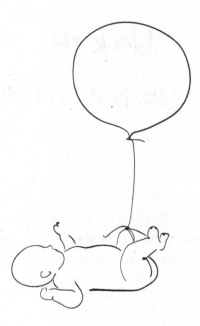

How to Do It

- Get four high-contrast balloons. Lay your baby on their back on a cushioned surface like a rug or play mat.
- Tie two loosely on baby's wrists.
- Tie two loosely on baby's ankles.
- Watch the fun begin as they move and shake their legs.

My Notes

_____
_____
_____
_____

Hack #14

Sit Up, Not Spit Up

It's important to remember that every baby develops at their own pace. While some babies may be able to sit up independently as early as 5–6 months old, others may not be able to do so until they are closer to 9 months old. Here's how to help them along.

Why It Works

Early baby exercises and milestones will help your baby gain the strength to sit up on their own. A recent study also showed that babies who can sit up unsupported are better able to learn about objects.

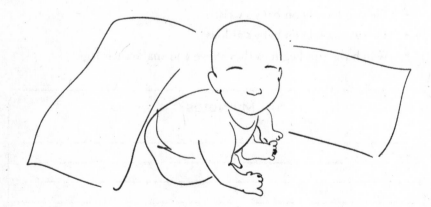

Tips

- While Bumbo-type seats are great for occasional use, don't over rely on these or use for more than 10 minutes at a time.
- Make sure your baby has strong neck and trunk control before trying to help them sit up.
- If your baby starts to cry or seems uncomfortable when sitting, pause the exercise and try again later.

How to Do It

- Sit on the floor on a comfortable rug or pad and cross your legs.
- Place your baby on the floor in a seated position right where your legs cross.
- Hold them at the hips to help them balance themselves.
- Place pillows around baby and prop them up. This will help them improve their balance to sit unsupported.

My Notes

_____

_____

_____

_____

_____

_____

_____

_____

Hack #15

Happy Baby

Many of us parents are already aware of the Happy Baby yoga pose through practicing in our own yoga classes. But did you know that this is a very beneficial exercise for baby? While most babies will start doing this on their own at 4–5 months, you can start them off early. Here's how to encourage this pose.

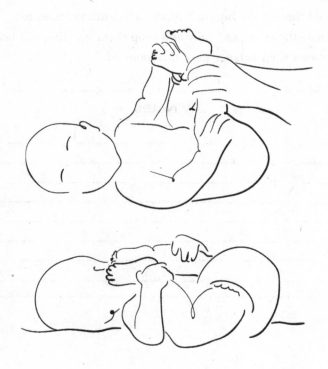

Why It Works

The Happy Baby pose is a relaxing, restorative pose that stretches the inner thighs, hips, groin, and hamstring muscles.

Tips

- Encourage this position by doing the same pose next to them and watch your baby try to mimic you.
- Place a rolled-up towel under your baby's back for additional support.

How to Do It

- Lay your baby down on a soft mat or rug.
- Draw your baby's knees up and pull their knees toward their chest.
- Place their hands on top of their feet and rock them gently.

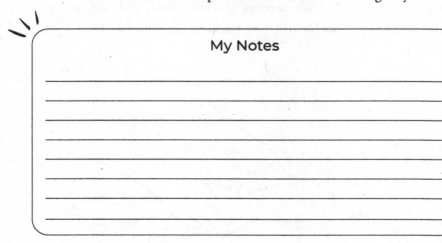

My Notes

Hack #16

The Roll Over

While it may seem like rolling should come easily, a lot of babies have a hard time mastering this skill that is so important for them when they are sleeping or preparing to sit and crawl. This milestone usually happens at 3–6 months. Here's how you can encourage rolling.

Why It Works

Rolling exercises help with developing trunk, head, and core strength, which are all important for achieving the bigger gross motor skills.

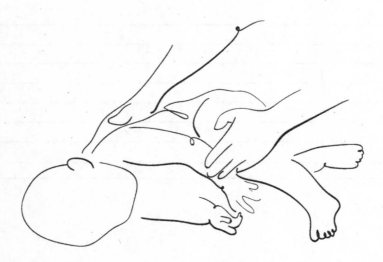

Tips

- Do not force baby to roll.
- Gently guide them and let their natural momentum take over.
- If your baby starts to cry or seems uncomfortable when rolling, pause the exercise and try again later.

How to Do It

- Lay your baby on their back on a soft surface such as a rug or play mat.
- Place your hands on their hips.
- Gently guide their left thigh to their right side, allowing their body to follow along naturally.
- Return to the center and repeat on the other side.

My Notes

_____

_____

_____

_____

_____

_____

_____

Hack #17

Pillow Play

Once your baby shows signs of sitting up and crawling, it's time you put their crawling skills to the test with a little soft pillow play. Just place five to ten pillows around your baby and watch them navigate the cushy obstacle course.

Why It Works

This activity helps your baby exercise all their muscles and facilitates coordination of their hands and legs. It is also very helpful for balance.

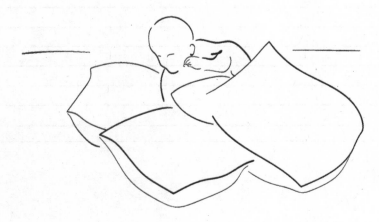

Tips

- Always supervise baby during this activity to make sure they are ready developmentally.
- Once your baby is able to navigate the floor pillows easily, try stacking some pillows to challenge them further.

How to Do It

- Once your baby is sitting up unassisted, place them on a soft rug or mat.
- Arrange five to ten pillows around them.
- Encourage them to start crawling around and over the pillows by placing a favorite toy out of reach.

My Notes

_____

_____

_____

_____

_____

_____

_____

Hack #18

A Helping Foot

For some reason, walking milestones have a tendency to throw even the most even-tempered parents into a tizzy. Most babies start walking between 9 and 18 months of age—that's a big range of normal. Take it from someone whose kids did not walk until 15 and 17 months, respectively: There's usually nothing to worry about, and just about all babies will at some point walk over to the fridge to steal your best snacks or walk over to the couch to hijack the TV remote. That said, developmental delays can and will happen, so if you want to give your baby a boost in the walking department, here is an exercise you can work on at home.

Why It Works

Holding your baby at the armpits or ribcage prevents them from tilting forward and allows their feet to have full contact with the floor, which helps them develop the strength and balance they need to walk.

Tips

- Don't pressure your baby to walk.
- Encourage and praise their efforts to stand or balance.
- Jumpers seem like they will help baby walk faster, but they are actually not good for your baby's development.
- If your child is not walking by 18–23 months, it's important to visit a physical therapist or speak to your pediatrician.

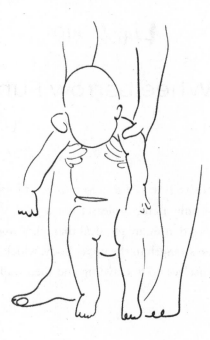

How to Do It

- Once your baby reaches 8 months and has good head control, let them cruise on the furniture by propping them up, holding their hand to assist, and letting them lean on furniture.
- Assist their walking by holding them right under the armpits or on their ribcage instead of at the fingertips.

My Notes

_____

_____

_____

_____

Hack #19

Wheelbarrow Fun

If you've ever played this fun backyard activity relay game, you'll know it's not only a crowd-pleaser but a great workout as well. It's also a popular activity that many physical therapists work on with their little clients to build up strength in the upper body, which will help your baby eventually pull themselves up to crawling and then walking.

Why It Works

Not only does this exercise strengthen your baby's shoulders and arm muscles, it also helps them learn balance, which will help with other motor skills activities.

Tips

- Start this activity at 6 months once your baby has firm head control.
- Always support baby at the hip joints and have a secure grip before lifting their lower half up.
- Make sure not to lift your baby too high or pitch them forward as they may not be ready developmentally. Start low and slow.
- Stop if your baby seems tired or irritable.

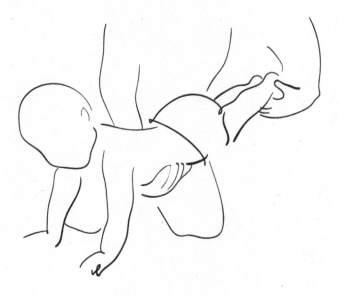

How to Do It

- Find a soft surface like a Toki mat (my favorite), a plush rug, or a spot to sit outside on the grass.
- Lay your baby on their belly and lift them up from the hips.
- Gently hold them and encourage them to start balancing on their hands, loosening your grip ever so slightly while they master balancing.

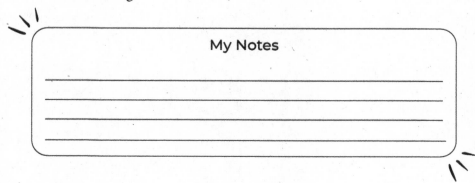

My Notes

Conclusion

Here we are at the end of the book, but you're only at the beginning of your journey with your wonderfully captivating, ever-changing baby. It's my hope that the more you use the ideas in this book, the more you will feel like an expert in all things natural baby care and be empowered in your role as a parent. While this book won't answer every single one of your questions (kids do have a way of surprising us when we least expect it!), the techniques and hacks included here should provide you with a strong foundation for caring for your growing child.

Incorporating baby massage and natural nurturing techniques into your everyday routine goes far beyond just the practical implications of physical wellness. By doing massage every day with your child, you'll be far more capable and more knowledgeable about your baby than when you started. Moreover, the techniques and massage practice you start today will lead to a whole host of benefits that you may not even foresee right now.

Connection is a big one. A study out of Princeton University followed 14,000 US children, and found that 40 percent lacked strong emotional bonds with their parents. The report found that kids ages 3 and under who fail to form a strong connection with parents are more likely to grow defiant, aggressive, and hyperactive as they get older. Babies who are massaged and interacted with frequently feel closer to their parents and become less aggressive. They also grow up to become more intelligent and can process information better than non-massaged peers.

What's more, your feeling of confidence and competence with handling your baby will significantly improve . . . and that's really 90 percent of the battle. Study after study shows that parents who massage their children regularly reported much higher satisfaction scores about being a parent and felt closer and more bonded to their baby. By practicing massage consistently with your baby, you will actually be teaching yourself the mindset you need to take on any challenge, issue, and developmental stage as your child blossoms into adulthood. You will be cultivating an attitude that is all about staying calm, present, and centered in the face of stress and tuning in to your child's needs so you can help them cope with life's many challenges. The confidence you'll get that you can handle anything life or your baby throws at you is a big bonus, for you and for baby.

I thank you for taking this journey with me and hope that this book has impressed upon you the importance of staying present. While babies can seem foreign, cranky, and unpredictable, having a regular massage practice helps you learn that you can tackle any challenge and learn to communicate with your baby even when they can't directly talk to you.

As parents, the one thing we know for sure in life is that everything changes, constantly. As soon as you master one stage with your child, you will need to acclimate to a completely different set of guidelines. In the end, it's this daily focused interaction with your child that helps you connect with them at whatever stage they are in and surrender to the way things are rather than what we would like them to be. You'll learn so much about your baby, yourself, and your limitless capacity to love another human being unconditionally . . . and that's the most priceless gift of all.

Acknowledgments

Thank you to everyone on the BenBella team who helped bring this book to life. Leah Wilson for giving me the green light and championing the project. A special thank-you to my tireless editor, Claire Schulz, who whipped the copy into shape and worked tirelessly to organize, refine, and streamline the manuscript.

I would like to also thank my talented illustrator, Dasha Kurinna, who brought my vision to life. A special thank-you to everyone working with me on growing the Kahlmi company, Adel Babataher and my wonderful team there.

Finally, a big thank-you to all my dear friends and family, my husband, Jay; sister, Leah; and my mother, Mira, who put up with me during my long hours of reclusive writing.

Selected Bibliography

Bahrami, Hamid, Mohammad Ali Kiani, and Mohammadreza Noras. "Massage for Infantile Colic: Review and Literature." *International Journal of Pediatrics* 4, no. 6 (2016): 1953–1958.

Çaka, Sinem Yalnızoğlu, and Duygu Gözen. "Effects of Swaddled and Traditional Tub Bathing Methods on Crying and Physiological Responses of Newborns." *Journal for Specialists in Pediatric Nursing* 23, no. 1 (January 2018): e12202. https://doi.org/10.1111/jspn.12202.

Choi, HyeJeong, Shin-Jeong Kim, Jina Oh, Myung-Nam Lee, SungHee Kim, and Kyung-Ah Kang. "The Effects of Massage Therapy on Physical Growth and Gastrointestinal Function in Premature Infants: A Pilot Study." *Journal of Child Health Care* 20, no. 3 (September 2016): 394–404. https://doi.org/10.1177/1367493515598647.

Cordero, María José Aguilar, Norma Mur Villar, Rafael Guisado Barrilao, Manuel Eduardo Cortés Cortés, and Antonio Manuel Sánchez López. "Application of Extra Virgin Olive Oil to Prevent Nipple Cracking in Lactating Women." *Worldviews on Evidence-Based Nursing* 12, no. 6 (December 2015): 364–369. https://doi.org/10.1111/wvn.12113.

Dalili, Hosein, Sanaz Sheikhi, Mamak Shariat, and Edith Haghnazarian. "Effects of Baby Massage on Neonatal Jaundice in Healthy Iranian

Infants: A Pilot Study." *Infant Behavior and Development* 42 (February 2016): 22–26. https://doi.org/10.1016/j.infbeh.2015.10.009.

Darmstadt, Gary L., Naila Z. Khan, Summer Rosenstock, Humaira Muslima, Monowara Parveen, Wajeeha Mahmood, A. S. M. Nawshad Uddin Ahmed, M. A. K. Azad Chowdhury, Scott Zeger, and Samir K. Saha. "Impact of Emollient Therapy for Preterm Infants in the Neonatal Period on Child Neurodevelopment in Bangladesh: An Observational Cohort Study." *Journal of Health, Population and Nutrition* 40 (2021): 24. https://doi.org/10.1186/s41043-021-00248-9.

Edraki, Mitra, Maryam Paran, Sedigheh Montaseri, Mostajab Razavi Nejad, and Zohre Montaseri. "Comparing the Effects of Swaddled and Conventional Bathing Methods on Body Temperature and Crying Duration in Premature Infants: A Randomized Clinical Trial." *Journal of Caring Sciences* 3, no. 2 (2014): 83–91. https://doi.org/10.5681/jcs.2014.009.

Ferber, Sari Goldstein, Moshe London, Jacob Kuint, Aron Weller, and Nava Zisapel. "Massage Therapy by Mothers Enhances the Adjustment of Circadian Rhythms to the Nocturnal Period in Full-Term Infants." *Journal of Developmental & Behavioral Pediatrics* 23, no. 6 (December 2002): 410–415. https://doi.org/10.1097/00004703-200212000-00003.

Fidler, Heidi. "Report Brief on a Maternal Massage Therapy Intervention and Neurodevelopmental Outcomes at 2 Years Corrected Age." *Advances in Neonatal Care* 10, no. 2 (April 2010): 98–99. https://doi.org/10.1097/ANC.0b013e3181d5e33e.

Field, Tiffany, and Maria Hernandez-Reif. "Sleep Problems in Infants Decrease Following Massage Therapy." *Early Child Development and Care* 168, no. 1 (2001): 95–104. https://doi.org/10.1080/0300443011680106.

Field, Tiffany, Miguel A. Diego, Maria Hernandez-Reif, Osvelia Deeds, and Barbara Figuereido. "Moderate Versus Light Pressure Massage Therapy Leads to Greater Weight Gain in Preterm Infants." *Infant Behavior and Development* 29, no. 4 (December 2006): 574–578. https://doi.org/10.1016/j.infbeh.2006.07.011.

Guzzetta, Andrea, Maria G. D'Acunto, Marco Carotenuto, Nicoletta Berardi, Ada Bancale, Enrico Biagioni, Antonio Boldrini, Paolo Ghirri, Lamberto Maffei, and Giovanni Cioni. "The Effects of Preterm Infant Massage on Brain Electrical Activity." *Developmental Medicine & Child Neurology* 53, no. 24 (September 2011): 46–51. https://doi.org/10.1111/j.1469-8749.2011.04065.x.

Hernandez-Reif, Maria, Miguel Diego, and Tiffany Field. "Preterm Infants Show Reduced Stress Behaviors and Activity After 5 Days of Massage Therapy." *Infant Behavior and Development* 30, no. 4 (December 2007): 557–561. https://doi.org/10.1016/j.infbeh.2007.04.002.

Liu, Zhi, Li Gang, Ma Yunwei, and Ling Lin. "Clinical Efficacy of Infantile Massage in the Treatment of Infant Functional Constipation: A Meta-Analysis." *Frontiers in Public Health* (2021): 9:663581. https://doi.org/10.3389/fpubh.2021.663581.

Ohmura, Nami, Lana Okuma, Anna Truzzi, Kazutaka Shinozuka, Atsuko Saito, Susumu Yokota, Andrea Bizzego, Eri Miyazawa, Masaki Shimizu, Gianluca Esposito, and Kumi O. Kuroda, "A Method to Soothe and Promote Sleep in Crying Infants Utilizing the Transport Response." *Current Biology* 32, no. 20 (2022): 4521–4529.e4. https://doi.org/10.1016/j.cub.2022.08.041.

Sezici, Emel, and Deniz Yigit. "Comparison Between Swinging and Playing of White Noise Among Colicky Babies: A Paired Randomised Controlled Trial." *Journal of Clinical Nursing* 27, no 3–4 (February 2018): 593–600. https://doi.org/10.1111/jocn.13928.

About the Author

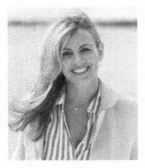

Elina Furman is a certified infant massage instructor with over 15 years in the baby industry. As the founder of Kahlmi, the first baby massager and wellness brand for families, she spends her days on social media helping anxious new moms navigate all the issues, questions, and freak-outs that having a new baby entails. While she may seem to know everything and anything about babies, Elina was actually a frazzled, mostly clueless first-time mom. She first became interested in baby massage having gone through colic with her oldest son and learning the art of child massage. Her work as a baby massage product inventor has won her awards from the Juvenile Product Manufacturing Association, the Baby Innovation Awards, and a Best of Seal from Pampers. She has appeared on countless TV shows and magazines to educate parents about the importance of baby massage. Born in Kiev, Ukraine, she lives in Connecticut with her husband and two sons.